Yoga
and Naturopathy
for Women

The Secret
Benefits of

Yoga
and Naturopathy
for Women

Parvesh Handa

Sterling Paperbacks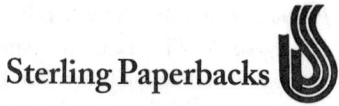

STERLING PAPERBACKS
An imprint of
Sterling Publishers (P) Ltd.
A-59, Okhla Industrial Area, Phase-II,
New Delhi-110020.
Tel: 26387070, 26386209; Fax: 91-11-26383788
E-mail: sterlingpublishers@airtelbroadband.in
ghai@nde.vsnl.net.in
www.sterlingpublishers.com

The Secret Benefits of
Yoga and Naturopathy for Women

© 2007, Parvesh Handa

ISBN 978- 81-207-3514-9

Published by Sterling Publishers Pvt. Ltd., New Delhi-110020.
Lasertypeset by Vikash Compographics, New Delhi.
Printed at Sterling Publishers Pvt. Ltd., New Delhi-110020

Advising Experts

Dr. D.S. Jaspal
Patron/President, Indian Medical Association, Haryana

Dr. Rita
Chairperson IMA, Haryana

Dr. Sarita Gupta, MD (obst & gynae)

Dr. Rajeev Gupta, MD (Radiology)
PGIMS Rohtak

Contents

Every Woman
Must be Aware of

Menstrual Disorders

Early Periods

Sometimes, periods start early in girls between the age of 10 and 11 due to hormonal imbalance in the body. It has been observed that in few cases, periods among teenage girls do not stop until hormones are administered when their haemoglobin level starts decreasing drastically. Due to continuous intake of hormones, there are chances to put on a lot of weight. Pelvic examination by sonography is essential in such conditions. The patient should be given iron supplements to combat anaemia and efforts should be taken to lose weight as obesity may further contribute to hormonal imbalance.

Recommended yogic exercises for all menstrual disorders are *dhanurasana, sirshasana, halasana, matsyasana, sarvangasana, shirshasana, salambha shirshasana* and *malasana*.

Amenorrhoea

Scanty discharge of menstrual blood or absence of menstrual flow may be due to anaemia, ill-health and imperfect development or functioning of the ovaries. Sudden fright or grief may also cause stoppage of the menstrual flow for months.

Steep 1 tablespoon each of sesame seeds and small caltrops (*gokhru*) in 200 ml water and grind them. Sweeten with sugar or honey and drink it. Do not overstrain yourself mentally or physically. Hot and cold hip bath and sunbathing is beneficial.

Dysmenorrhoea

The symptoms in this case include pain during menstruation, nausea and feeling of weakness generally due to inflammation of the internal organs, e.g. the womb, ovary defects or malfunctioning of the fallopian tubes.

The leaves of the herbs–Indian wild pepper (*sambhalu*), horse radish (*sahinjana*), Indian lilac (*bakayan*), wild chicory (*kasni*), black night-shade (*mako*), marshmallow (*khatmi*), cotton plant (*narm kapas*) and dill (*soya*) should be boiled in water. Later they should be cooked in sesame oil, dried and tied on the lower abdomen like a poultice. Most of the herbs are available at leading herbal stores in big towns.

Menorrhagia

It is the excessive discharge of blood from the womb during periods usually due to faulty functioning of the ovaries.

Have the powder of dried amla with milk. A hot and cold hip bath is very beneficial for menorrhagia patients.

4-D Ultrasound

A 4-D ultrasound is the latest addition in the armamentarium of an obstetrician. A 3-D ultrasound gives a three dimensional view of the baby in the womb.

An ultrasound gives a two dimensional view, which makes the diagnosis of the malformations. The surface of the body of the baby and internal malformations can be visualised clearly. A 3-D ultrasound is like a still photograph whereas a 4-D ultrasound is like taking video film of the foetus malformation and the pregnancy, especially in case the mother is over the age of 35 years and has delivered a malformed baby in the past.

Rashes or Pain in the Breasts

Rashes on the breasts can be due to various reasons. The most common cause is allergy due to synthetic brassière or bacterial, viral or fungal infection. A mammogram or an ultrasound is done in case of lumpy and painful breasts. If there is a cyst in the breasts then you can take any analgesic and wear tight bras to support them and to relieve the pain. 400mg of vitamin E or B taken over a period of time may lessen the pain. If the pain is severe, danazol or hormone therapy is recommended. Periodic examination of the breasts is also necessary.

Effect of Copper-T

Insertion of the Copper-T for family planning can lead to a change in the menstrual flow for a couple of months. Some women experience backache, white discharge from the vagina, heavy menstrual discharge and congestion and irritation around the cervix.

Stretch Marks

Stretch marks on the abdomen and the stomach are common in women generally after the delivery of the child. Striae gravidarum or stretch marks appear on the lower abdomen in 50 to 90 percent of all pregnant women usually in the later half of the pregnancy. These may also appear on thighs, hips, buttocks, breasts and the upper arms of women, which appear as pinkish lines on fair complexioned women and lighter than the normal skin in dark complexioned women. The market is flushed with creams and ointments to cure these stretch marks. The stretch marks depend upon the family history, weight gained and the nutritional status of women.

Recommended yogic exercises include *ardh chandrasana, dhanurasana, ourdhva paschimottanasana, paschimottanasana, uddyana bandhasana, pawanmuktasana, utthita padmasana, janusirasana and parivritta janusirasana.*

Cramps before Periods

Between 30% to 50% women suffer cramps during or before menses, which differs from woman to woman . Persistent night cramps are often caused by poor blood circulation. The cramps felt in the abdomen before menses are difficult to cope. But that doesn't indicate any abnormality in the genitals of the woman. About 10% women have severe pain and cramps during menses and are even unable to walk due to stress and strain as in the case of the delivery of the child. During menstruation the pain in the lower back and pelvis is common and is called 'initial pain'. The main reason for such pain is hormonal changes generally as a result of the contraction of uterus when it discharges blood. Yogic exercises stimulating the nerves of the affected parts of the legs relieve cramps. There are several natural remedies to cure this painful disorder as below:

- Add 7 drops of the essential oil of cloves (aromatic spicy herb) to a teaspoon of sunflower oil and massage the muscles of the affected area.

- Tincture of myrrh rubbed directly into the affected muscle, gives quick relief.

- Mix two drops each of the essential oils of lemon, pine and juniper with 1 tablespoon of sunflower oil. Massage the body with this oil.

In case of cramps before periods a hot water bath of the lower part of the abdomen relieves pain. Consult a doctor if the pain is severe and doesn't stop for a few days. This pain is different from the menstrual pain or a pain experienced during and after intercourse. Smoking, sleeplessness and the intake of carbohydrates and fatty foods can cause severe cramps. Bad sitting postures, frequent headache, diarrhoea, constipation, nausea or pain prior to menstruation further worsen the condition. A regular practice of yogic exercises benefit.

Gomukhasana (the cow head posture)

To practise this asana, sit on the floor folding the left leg against the right buttock and right leg over the left leg so that one knee lies over the other. Now take both the hands behind your back and interlock the fingers. Then interchange the position of your legs and arms. Hold this position for 10 to 15 counts each side.

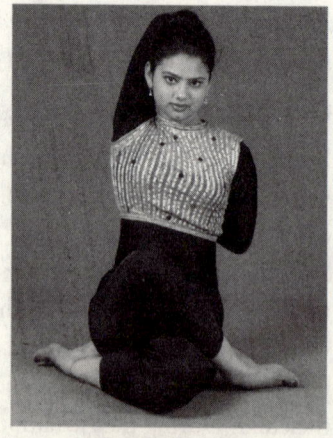

Gomukhasana

Benefits

1. Relieves cramps in the calves or feet that commonly occur during pregnancy while resting or sleeping.
2. Strengthens lungs and heart.
3. Relieves itching in the genital tract.
4. Helps in case of displacement of the uterus.
5. Relieves pain in the groin preceding the menses.
6. Restores the synovial fluid (a joint fluid in the body).
7. Strengthens the bones of the entire body.
8. This posture is very beneficial for the treatment of paralysis (palsy).

Morning Sex

Early morning is the best time to have sex due to the following reasons:

- The testosterone level in the male partner is higher in early morning hours.
- Men and women have higher levels of growth of the hormones due to increased energy after the restful night.
- Often a man awakes with a full bladder, which compresses the venous blood return and prevents the blood escaping from the penis. As a result the male partner experiences spontaneous erections in the morning.
- Sex during the night when the blood flow in the digestive system is predominant lacks pleasure. Good sex act requires good blood flow in the sex organs and is achieved better in the morning with empty stomach.

To enhance the pleasure of sexual intercourse, regular practice of yogic exercises such as *mandukasana, paschimottanasana, matsyasana, setubandha sarvangasana, supta vajrasana* and *natrajasana* leave good effects.

Leakage of Semen from the Vagina

The semen leaks out of the vagina after sexual intercourse, as a result women who are unable to conceive feel disappointed. Every woman should be aware that it is normal as a very small quantity of semen enters the uterus after the intercourse and rest of it has to come out of the vagina sooner or later. In fact, an inadequate sperm count in the semen may be the reason for not conceiving.

Ovary Cancer in Women

It is generally caused due to the rapid succession of childbirth resulting in wear and tear of the cervical tissues and natural genital secretions. The following symptoms are observed when the patient suffers from cervical cancer:

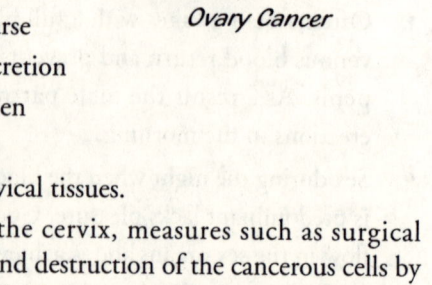

Ovary Cancer

- Abnormal blood stained vaginal discharge
- Intermittent prolonged menstrual bleeding
- Bleeding due to intercourse
- Foul smelling vaginal secretion
- Pain in the lower abdomen
- Constant backache
- Wear and tear of the cervical tissues.

To treat the cancer of the cervix, measures such as surgical removal of the affected part and destruction of the cancerous cells by radium or cobalt are adopted. If not treated at the initial stage the cancerous cells may spread to the liver and the brain.

Blood Tests for Women

A blood test can reveal various disorders in a woman's body. Every female from a pre-teen to one at the menopausal stage at some time or the other has to undergo a blood test on the recommendation of the doctor. The blood tests suggested for women are usually of six types:

- *CBC-ESR Test:* This test is required to find out the presence of an infection or an inflammatory reaction. The test may count red cells in the blood. A high white blood count reveals the dreaded cancer of the blood (leukemia).

- *Follicular Stimulating Hormones (FSH) Test:* This test is recommended to the teenage girls by the gynaecologist in case of irregular periods.

- *Haemogram Test:* Women with excessive bleeding are required to go for Haemogram test, which highlights the anaemic condition and also checks diabetes.

- *The Serum Beta (HCG) Test:* This test is carried out to confirm pregnancy and is recommended when the woman has missed her periods.

- *HIV Test:* It is important for every pregnant women to get herself examined for sexually transmitted diseases such as syphilis, gonorrhoea and hepatitis-B, to make the decision of whether to continue the pregnancy or not.

- *RH factor:* This test is essential for pregnant women. If the mother is RH negative (RH-) the baby is usually delivered through a caesarean procedure.

Loose Vaginal Muscles

Loose vaginal muscles are not a hindrance in satisfying the male partner. Recommended yogic postures are – *vajroli mudra, omkarasana, upavista konasana* and *salambha shirshasana.*

Benefits

- Help to tighten and strengthen loose vaginal muscles.
- Relieve the disorders of the pelvic region and strengthen all the sex organs among both sexes.
- Strengthen the anterior and posterior parts of the pubic muscles.

Vajroli mudra

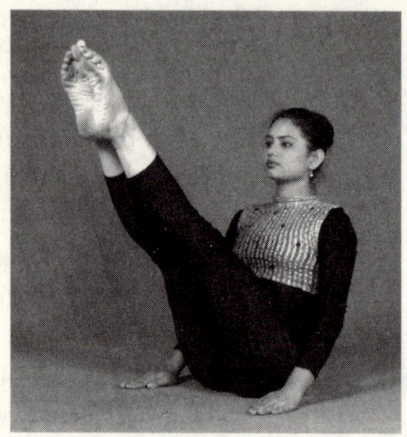

Sit in padmasana (lotus pose) or any comfortable meditative asana. Place hands on the knees, close the eyes, feel relaxed and breathe through the nose. After a deep inhalation, hold the breath and take your legs upwards, pulling and tensing the lower abdomen and contracting the pelvic muscles as if you have an urge to pass urine but wish to hold it for some time. Now exhale, relax and repeat the posture.

Vajroli mudra

Benefits

1. Strengthens the thighs and abdominal muscles.
2. Rids the digestive organs of toxins.
3. Helps develop will power.
4. Relieves pain in the lower belly before or during menstruation.
5. Helps to prevent premature ejaculation and delays the orgasm.

Functioning of the Aerola

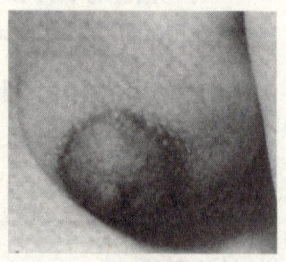

Many women want to know why their breasts are heavy as compared to men. Most of the women are ignorant about the functioning of their breasts. Aerola is the pigmented area surrounding the nipple. The size of the aerola varies considerably from woman to woman and from breast to breast. The aerola consists of several oil

Aerola

producing montromery's glands, which may form raised bumps and are sensitive to a woman's menstrual cycle. These glands protect and lubricate the nipples during lactation.

Preeclamptic Toxaemia

Preeclamptic Toxaemia (PET) is a combination of oedema (e.g. swelling on the ankles and fingers followed by puffiness of the face with increased blood pressure and presence of protein in the urine). Obese women and teenage girls are usually seen suffering from this disorder. Women with a family history of high blood pressure are prone to the risk. In case it is not treated timely it may cause fits and the birth of a retarded child due to infra-uterine growth affecting the growth of the infant in the womb. The disease is more common in anaemic and malnourished women. For the healthy growth of an unborn baby, it is important for the females to abstain from smoking cigarettes and consuming alcohol. Certain conditions like high blood pressure, chronic kidney diseases, heart ailments and some infections also affect the baby's growth.

Recommended yogic exercises are – *pranayama, paschimottanasana, ardha matsyendrasana, sarvangasana* and *shavasana.*

Abortion

Women with unwanted pregnancies always resort to abortion. With restricted law imposed by the Government, an abortion is illegal. Unwanted pregnancy may be due to the following reasons:

- Contraceptive failure
- Too much shyness to discuss contraception with the male partner, because of which a female becomes pregnant.
- Urge to have sex with the opposite sex in youth without thinking about its after-effects.

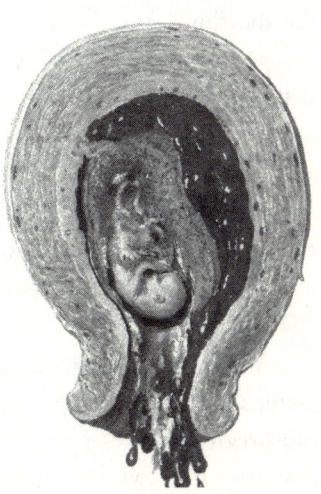

Inevitable abortion

• Unawareness about the contraceptive methods.

Most abortions are carried out before 12 weeks of pregnancy and by the common method called vacuum aspiration or suction. The cervix is dilated or widened carefully and the contents of the womb are sucked out using a suction apparatus.

Another method of abortion, instead of vacuum aspiration between 12 to 14 weeks of pregnancy is dilation and curettage by inserting prostaglandin pessaries (a thimble -like fine rubber cervical cap about 15 cm long, which looks like a condom used by males, can be pushed into the vagina to cover the external genitalia and uterine mouth prior to coitus and should be slipped out 5 to 6 hours after the intercourse. The use of pessary combined with a spermicidal cream is more effective. Another substance called laminaria is also inserted into the vagina to avoid pregnancy.

The contents of the womb are removed by an instrument called a curette made of soft wire rather than by section. It cleans the womb and most of the tissues removed during abortion look like a very heavy menstrual discharge. If the bleeding persists and is very heavy, consult a doctor immediately. Retained products in the uterus lead to an infection. This sometimes happen about a week or ten days after the abortion.

Abortion after 12 weeks becomes more difficult although it is still safe. In this process, after dilating the cervix, the doctor may insert instruments into the womb. This technique is called dilation and evacuation and is carried out under general anaesthetic. Late abortions are conducted by hysterectomy, a technique used very rarely, which involves removing the contents of the womb in an operation very much like a caesarean section. It is done under general anaesthetic.

Any abortion conducted after 12 weeks is likely to cause pain and cramps, which may last several days and the womb shrinks back to its pre-pregnancy size. The bleeding goes on for about a week. Avoid activities like swimming, taking a hot bath, wearing tampon or having sexual intercourse for six weeks.

A regular practice of yogic exercises to strengthen the reproductive organs makes the pregnancy strong and the foetus healthy. In a premature delivery, usually the infant is delivered in the eighth month and has the risk of survival. This is due to the weakness of the cervical muscles, which support the uterus in expectant mothers. Yogic exercises, which strengthen the reproductive organs are – *sarvangasana, paschimottanasana* and *supta vajrasana.*

Breast Care

Here are some do's and don'ts about breast care and breastfeeding:

- Keep the nipples clean and dry to prevent them from becoming sore and infected. Do not apply soap on the nipples and aerola to avoid cracks.

- Wash the breasts and nipples with water to remove the traces of milk.

- Make sure to change the bra frequently. The secretion of nipples causes infection.

- In case nipples are not soft and supple, apply some cream or oil. Avoid the use of mustard oil, as it irritates. Keep the breasts exposed to air for sometime in a day.

- Breasts sag if the infant suckles while sitting or reclining in a faulty posture. Always let the baby suckle in a sitting position with the child in the lap and mother's hands under the head.

- Remove the remaining milk after feeding the child.

Recommended yogic exercises to enhance the beauty of breast, to prevent them from sagging and to reshape them if underdeveloped are – *bhujangasana, dhanurasana, chakrasana* and *pawanmuktasana.*

Mother's milk is the most perfectly balanced food that a baby needs for growth during the first 3-4 months. It prevents many illnesses, infections and allergies. Lactation helps in controlling the bleeding after the delivery, the womb returns to its normal position, extra weight gained during the pregnancy is lost, prevents cancer and helps in spacing children. Breastfeeding is very convenient for mothers during travelling. Mother's milk is easily digestible as compared to cow's milk.

Bhujangasana (the cobra posture)

Lie on your stomach joining legs and place the palms on sides. Taking the support of the arms slowly raise the head and the trunk. Lean backwards as much as possible without raising the abdominal portion from the ground. Hold for 6-8 seconds and gradually return to the starting position. Repeat this exercise 3-4 times.

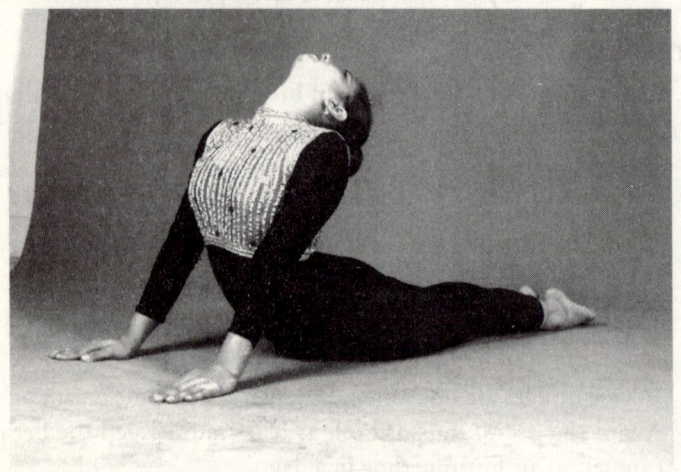

Bhujangasana

Benefits

* This posture soothes backache, stimulates digestion, leaves a beneficial effect on the kidneys (adrenal glands).
* Strengthens breast muscles, corrects menstrual problems.
* Cures constipation, indigestion, dysentery, wind trouble and abdominal disorders.

Dhanurasana (the bow posture)

Lie flat on the stomach keeping the arms stretched on both sides. Raise the head and the upper part of the body. Bend the knees and hold the ankles with the hands. Tense the arch muscles and arch the back. Remain in this position as long as you can comfortably. Return to the initial position, rest and repeat.

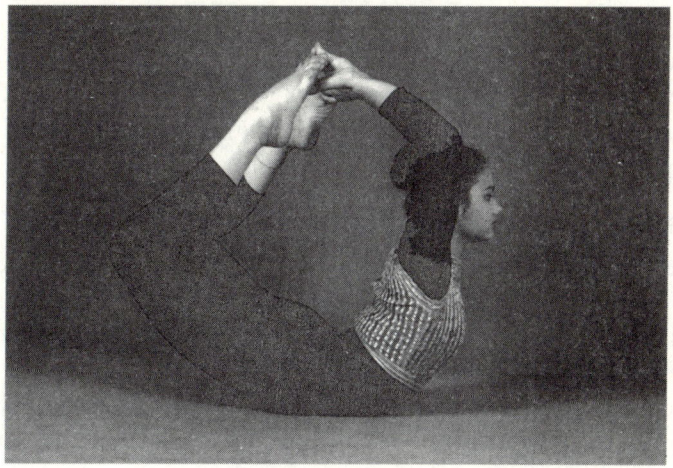

Dhanurasana

Benefits

- Tones up the muscles of the abdominal organs, spinal cord, lungs and chest.
- Cures irregular or faulty menstruation in women, stimulates the endocrine glands and prevents fat from forming around the stomach and hips.
- Leaves beneficial effect on the adrenal glands, thyroid, parathyroid, pituitary and sex glands.
- Relieves extra fat around the stomach, waist, hips and thighs.
- Helps in the development of breasts.

Lesbianism

A lesbian is a female homosexual. Rather than being sexually attracted to the opposite sex, sometimes a woman is sexually attracted to her own sex.

Puerperium

It is a medical term for the post delivery period when the genital passage and the uterus gradually get back to the original size. The complete involution of the uterus takes about six weeks. Vaginal discharge, which is initially pale pink "fleshy" blood with mucous gradually becomes lighter in colour till it finally stops. During puerperium, there is a chance of the uterus getting infected. A thorough hygiene has to be maintained with a light nutritious diet supported with adequate vitamins and minerals.

Displacement of the Uterus

The uterus or the womb is slung in the pelvic cavity and has sufficient movement in all directions. However, its natural position is upwards and forwards between the bladder and the rectum. The displacement of the uterus occurs because of several reasons and is usually accompanied by inflammation. The downward displacement of the uterus is known as prolapse. In this condition the uterus slips downwards in the space between the bladder and the rectum. This condition is more common in older women.

The uterus gets distend during pregnancy when the foetus grows. The muscles supporting the uterus must be strong enough to bear the burden of the growing child in it. After the delivery of the child the uterus and the surrounding muscles get back to their former shape and size. The symptoms, which indicate the displacement of the uterus include backache or headache and heaviness in the bowels. Nerve centres are badly affected due to the displacement of the uterus. The patient may be irritable and feel depressed. Doctors generally advise surgical interference for the treatment.

A healthy woman doesn't experience any difficulty in childbirth and there are no complications even afterwards. Remember, prenatal care and proper diet can ward off the danger of displacement of the uterus. If the patient is weak and old, it could take long to put the displaced uterus back in shape. The following natural steps are recommended:

- Take to fasting. Fasting should be continued for at least three days.
- Have a good diet containing enough fruits, milk and green vegetables.
- Proper rest and relaxation drain out tension from the body.

- Have a regular exercise plan designed to tone up the muscles supporting the uterus. Also seek advise of a naturopath.
- Rub the parts immersed in water vigorously while having hip bath.
- Keep a hard pillow under the buttocks instead of under the head. This will help the uterus to return to its initial position.
- Lie on the floor with your knees touching your breast.
- Lie down after a meal with a pillow under your back.

Recommended yogic exercises are – *pawanmuktasana, gomukhasana, sarvangasana, shallabhasana, matsyasana, halasana* and *viparitakarniasana.*

Premenstrual Syndrome

Some women have mild to moderate discomfort a few days before or during menstruation. A few have severe symptoms of distress that may include – fatigue, depression, anxiety, body swelling, headache, pain in the thighs, back, or abdomen. Premenstrual syndrome, a disorder characterised by some or all of these symptoms, may occur when progesterone levels are inadequate. The following natural remedies are recommended:

- Put ¼ teaspoon of sea salt in a cup of warm water and drink. This will stop your sugar craving.
- Keep eating after short intervals.
- Drink ginger tea, which helps cure fatigue.

Female Hormones

Female hormones – estrogen and progesterone are produced in the ovaries by the pituitary gland, the master endocrine gland of the body, which gives the woman strength, stamina, graceful curves and a feminine shape. Estrogen, the prominent female hormone provides enormous drive, energy and power. When a girl reaches eleven or twelve years of age, her ovaries start producing large quantities of estrogen causing her to grow and develop rapidly. The next 35 years are the reproductive years of a woman's life when she can conceive and produce children. Progesterone has a special function of its own.

Progesterone, which is produced by the ovaries prepares the uterine wall so that the implantation of the fertilised egg may occur.

Excessive Sexual Urge in Women

There are women who are extremely passionate and feel an uncontrolled desire for sex. They are constantly attracted towards the opposite sex. This is often due to the following reasons:

- Deep sense of insecurity produced by neglect in childhood and adolescence.
- Genetically, some females are hyper-fertile and highly sexual.

Women with excessive desire for sex need psychotherapy. Hormone therapy neutralises the effect of estrogen by administering progesterone hormones, which help to a large extent.

Sex after Menopause

Menopause is not the end of sex life and a woman can continue having normal sex for years after that also. Many women enjoy satisfying sexual partnership even in old age. There are numerous couples in 60s who are involved in active sex life. Sometimes, menopausal women face problems having sex due to severe dryness of the genital organs. As a result they experience pain during intercourse. Lubricating creams or estrogen ointments help to prevent the rapid atrophy of the vaginal mucosa.

Recommended yogic exercises are – *trikonasana, ardh sarvangasana, parivritta janusirasana, garudasana, vir bhadraasana, ek pada uttanasana, tarasana* and *hasta parshavasana.*

Fungal Infections

Occasionally, the female genital organs get infected with fungus. This may sometimes occur during pregnancy because of the increased sugar content of the blood. Women suffering from diabetes are more likely to have fungal infections, which may result in intense itching around the genitals and a thick discharge from the vagina. Any tendency towards diabetes should be corrected without delay. Take a warm vinegar douche once or twice a day, followed by insertion of Mycostatin in consultation with a doctor.

Heavy Menstrual Discharge

Regular monthly bleeding or menstruation occurs in all women from adolescence to menopause. Some women also have slight signs of blood on the day of ovulation and midway between the regular menstrual periods, which is not abnormal. Heavy vaginal bleeding during the childbearing age may be due to the following reasons:

- Miscarriage or abortion
- Ectopic pregnancy
- Malignant tumours of the uterus or cervix

Women with irregular or very heavy bleeding should have a Pap smear (test) done at least every six months in which small amount of material from the cervix is smeared on a glass slide and examined pathologically.

Intermittent spotting may be due to cervical polyp, a condition more common in women above forty years of age. Heavy bleeding may also be due to fibroid tumours and polyps in the uterus. In such cases either the tumour or perhaps the entire uterus should be removed. Endometriosis may also cause heavy or painful bleeding in younger women. Various other conditions, such as blood diseases, heart failure, alcoholism, cirrhosis of the liver, vitamin B deficiencies, and abnormality in either thyroid or pituitary or adrenal glands may result in heavy bleeding. The treatment depends on the cause.

- A bed rest is always advisable following heavy bleeding.
- The patient should be given a high protein diet and multivitamins.
- In case of heavy loss of blood, a transfusion may be needed.
- Heavy bleeding following the abortion usually requires a surgical operation to clean the uterus.
- Bleeding arising from tumours of the uterus and other pelvic organs may need to be controlled by surgery.
- If the woman is in her mid-pregnancy and suddenly begins to haemorrhage, she should be rushed to the hospital at once. All the products of conception should be expelled from the uterus, otherwise bleeding may not cease and there is danger of serious infection in the uterus.

Foreplay

Foreplay is the secret of sexual pleasure during intercourse. The sexual arousal of the partners is known as foreplay. To increase the woman's cooperation in sex, the male stimulates the erotic zones such as breast nipples, lips, face, neck, genitalia (especially the clitoris), thighs and back, which provide satisfying release to the women. Female orgasm is the acme of pleasure, associated with spontaneous spasms of the muscles in and around the genitalia. Such contractions come in waves and this sexual release of female corresponds to the climax experienced by the male partner at the time of ejaculation. Women attain an orgasmic spontaneous release through manual practice than through an intercourse, some others get an orgasmic spontaneous release during sleep (similar to night emissions in males). For most women sexual gratification is an overall feeling of satisfaction at the end of the act.

Fibroids (Leiomyoma)

It is the most common neoplasms of the uterus occurring in approximately 20 to 30% of females above the age of 30 years. These tumours are most common in dark complexioned women. They are usually multiple and are the commonest cause of enlargement of the non-pregnant uterus. A symptomatic pain and uterine bleeding may occur frequently in this disorder. Fibroids may be classified into three categories: intramural, submucosal and subserosal. Intramural fibroid is the most common among them.

Varicose Veins

Varicose veins are the enlarged and twisted veins just below the skin, usually in the legs. Due to increased pressure the veins lose elasticity and become elongated. Varicose veins have a bluish snake-like appearance.

As the blood returns to the heart it passes through special thin-walled channels called veins. These vessels swell as the blood builds up behind them. Blood flowing from the head and the upper chest flows downward towards the heart. On the other hand, blood coming from the lower extremities must flow upward. To make it possible, nature has provided valves in the veins so that blood can flow only towards the heart and never in the other direction. Constipation, smoking and hot baths are all contributory factors for varicose veins.

The varicose veins in the legs (especially around the ankles and valves) and thighs become enlarged and incompetent to prevent a backflow of blood resulting in stagnation and dilatation of the vessels, followed by swelling, pain, inflammation or phlebitis. If a person suffering from varicose veins keeps standing for a long time, it can lead to reduced blood supply to the muscles. Varicose veins seem to run in families. This ailment is more frequent in pregnancy and obesity due to increased pressure in the pelvis or abdomen, which slows down the flow of blood to the heart from the lower extremities. The following measures are suggested to treat varicose veins:

- Check the weight as every extra amount added to the weight increases the pressure on the venous circulation.
- Blood sugar should remain within the prescribed limits.
- Avoid prolonged standing.
- Wear comfortable padded low-heel shoes.
- Wear varicose vein stockings available at a chemist or a surgical store.
- A hot and cold foot bath before bed time improves circulation, prevents varicosities and helps the varicose veins to heal.
- Walking or jogging in water (in a swimming pool) is very helpful to relieve varicosity.
- Vitamin C strengthens the walls of the veins (recommended dose 2,000 to 3000 mg daily).
- Elderflower tea and Rosemary tea with honey are old-fashioned remedies to aid the circulation.
- Raise the legs several times a day and sleep with the foot of the bed raised six to eight inches higher than the head side.
- Massage the legs gently but do not scratch the varicose veins because varicose ulcers can develop from a sore place and can be very unpleasant. Excellent massage oils for varicose veins are

olive oil, sweet almond oil, essential oils of cypress, calendula, rosemary and lavender.

The signs of trouble include swelling along the course of the veins, followed by muscle cramps and a tired feeling of the calf muscles. Sometimes, the skin over the lower part of the leg may break-down forming a large, ugly painful ulcer, especially when thrombophlebitis develops. Surgery is the best treatment, especially when the large veins of the legs and the thighs are involved. However, regular practice of yoga relieves varicose veins and cramps.

Choosing Contraceptives

Newly weds are often ignorant about the right contraceptive. However, it is the personal decision of the couple to adopt a contraceptive method. The doctors often recommend few methods to suit an individual. For a newly married couple, the best options are condoms, spermicides and OCPs. In case of a woman who has never conceived before, using an intra-uterine device (IUD) could result in the infection of the fallopian tubes or the uterus, which may lead to infertility. The couple blessed with one child would like to space out the other. For them birth control pills are the best option, but these have to be taken daily. The permanent method of contraception is most recommended in case the couple doesn't want any more children. But it is prudent to wait till your child/children is about five years of age. So depending upon the economic background and the circumstances one should choose the right contraceptive. IUD prevents pregnancy by its copper action, thereby preventing embryo implantation in the uterus. On expiry, its copper contents get exhausted and its efficiency is decreased. Though the IUD itself can act as a foreign body and prevent pregnancy, it needs to be changed on its expiry. You should get the old one removed and the new one inserted within 5-7 days of your periods.

Most of the women are unaware of intra-uterine devices. It is an synthetic spiral or T-shaped tiny gadget that is fitted into the uterus. The device retards the passage of sperms into the uterus and prevents pregnancy. These are of various types like the spiral loop, copper T, and nova T with silver. Sometimes, the woman becomes pregnant despite the device when it slips. Frequent bleeding, heavy periods and infection are some of the common problems seen in women fitted with this device.

Female Orgasm

Female orgasm is the acme of pleasure associated with spontaneous spasm of muscles in and around the genitalia (mainly the clitoris and vagina). Such contractions come in waves and the sexual release of the female corresponds to the climax experienced by the male partner at the time of ejaculation. Many women attain an orgasmic release easily through manual practice than through an act of intercourse. Some others get an orgasmic spontaneous release during sleep as in case of night emission in males. For most women sexual gratification is an overall feeling of satisfaction at the end of the act. Recommended yogic exercises to enhance sexual power in such cases are *mandukasana, supta vajrasana, paschimottanasana, salambha shirshasana* and *parasarita pada uttanasana.*

Artificial Insemination

It is done with the husband or donor's sperm, around the time of the woman's ovulation. The sperms are injected into the cervical canal to make sure the sperms have found their way up to the uterus. A donor's sample is required to find out the vitality of the semen and the sperms.

2

Pregnancy and Post-natal Problems

Pregnancy Tests

Most of the pregnancy tests are based on the hormonal concentration of bHCG in urine. This test is sensitive and becomes positive as early as 2 to 3 days before a missed period due to pregnancy. The accuracy is 98.5%. Collect the early morning urine sample in a clean bottle. Only a few drops of urine are sufficient for a pregnancy test. 14 days after a missed period is the usual time to have a pregnancy test. A few doctors suggest hormone pills. Sometimes, a woman may bleed even if she is pregnant and this delays the detection of pregnancy.

Sex During Pregnancy

Having sexual intercourse during pregnancy does not harm the foetus. One can continue sexual intercourse right up to the onset of labour. As the abdomen enlarges, a woman may find intercourse more comfortable in positions that put less or absolutely no pressure on the abdomen like side-by-side or the female on the top. If a woman has complications like bleeding or pain in the abdomen, then she should refrain from sexual activities. Even nipple stimulation is to be avoided in such cases as it can induce pre-term labour.

Doctors often advise to avoid intercourse from 6th to 12th week of pregnancy as it can cause miscarriage. Sexual abstinence is recommended during the last two months of pregnancy too. At this time, there is risk of the essential amniotic fluid leakage during intercourse. However, the couple can and should engage in gentle love making, fondling and kissing. Intercourse during the first three months and the last two months of pregnancy is not advisable. During 4th to 7th month of pregnancy, intercourse is allowed unless there are medical reasons. Sexual acts such as oral and anal sex should be strictly avoided throughout the pregnancy.

Acidity During Pregnancy

Acidity, belching and flatulence occur during pregnancy because of the growing baby in the womb. The enlarging uterus occupies more and more space in the abdomen as a result of which the stomach is pushed up. This leads to a reflux of the acid present in the stomach and into the food pipe causing heartburn. Try taking small frequent meals so that the stomach is not very full. Avoid foods that cause acidity such as tea, coffee, colas and spicy and sour foods. Take dinner at least two hours before bedtime. To cure heartburn, take a glass of milk with honey.

Post-natal Depression

Depression is common among women, especially after childbirth, which causes them to lose sexual desire and other interests, besides feeling irritable and fatigued most of the time. Depression is more likely to occur if the woman feels isolated and if there is inadequate support from her husband and other members of her family. During the period of pregnancy, women should pay visits to the doctor for regular check ups between six and eight weeks and also post delivery, which gives them the opportunity to discuss all their problems. The following natural remedies are suggested:

- Sunlight: Body needs sunlight for its growth and development. The lack of sunlight can disturb the production of key hormones and brain chemicals, triggering depression.
- Exercise: Exercising is of utmost importance. An hour a day of exercise for a week is a universal prescription for people suffering from depression.
- Light music: Music lifts one's mood and keeps depression at bay.
- Yogic exercises : *Setubandha sarvangasana* is helpful to relieve depression.

Post-natal Sex

After childbirth, a woman's sexual desires and activities are conditioned on several factors as below:

• Strain of parenthood
• A painful episiotomy scar (vaginal cut, usually given at the time of delivery)

Sexual intercourse can be resumed whenever a woman feels comfortable about it. Women who breast-feed are usually more sexually aroused and responsive than women who choose to bottle-feed their babies. If intercourse continues to be painful, the doctor should be immediately consulted.

Post-natal Menstruation

If the mother is breastfeeding the baby, usually she doesn't menstruate for nearly six months. It has been observed that in approximately 20% to 25% cases, women start their periods within three months after the childbirth and about 30% to 50% women start to menstruate after three to four months and remaining after six to seven months. Ovulation is useful before the 20th week after the childbirth, but very few breastfeeding mothers ovulate before this period. However, pregnancy rarely occurs in the first four to five months of puerperium. A mother should continue breastfeeding, even if periods have started. Periods have no ill effects on the child and the quality of breast milk.

Post-natal Weight Reduction

A woman starts gaining weight during pregnancy, because the skin and muscles grow to hold the constant weight of the growing foetus in the womb. One shouldn't worry about this. The muscles gradually tighten up again after some time. Women should undertake exercises post-delivery. Breastfeeding helps the stomach to get back to shape as it helps the uterus to contract.

Sometimes, few days after the childbirth, the colour of the vaginal discharge changes from light yellowish to pale brown. Some women have a rush of blood when the baby starts breastfeeding. If you pass blood clots or fresh blood or the lochia (the normal vaginal discharge of blood and pus from the uterus) smells unpleasant, consult your doctor immediately. These are the signs of the part of placenta being left inside the womb or there could also be an infection. (After giving birth to a baby, women are often prone to infections). Make sure to keep the vaginal area clean and wash it with a mild soap and water after every trip to the toilet.

Surya Namaskar

Every type of yoga exercise helps to stimulate the nerves of a particular portion of the body, but the ten positions of *Surya Namaskar* (Sun Exercise), which involve bending forward and backward are especially helpful to slim the entire body. Surya Namaskar should be done with a relaxed body at least six to eight weeks after the delivery.

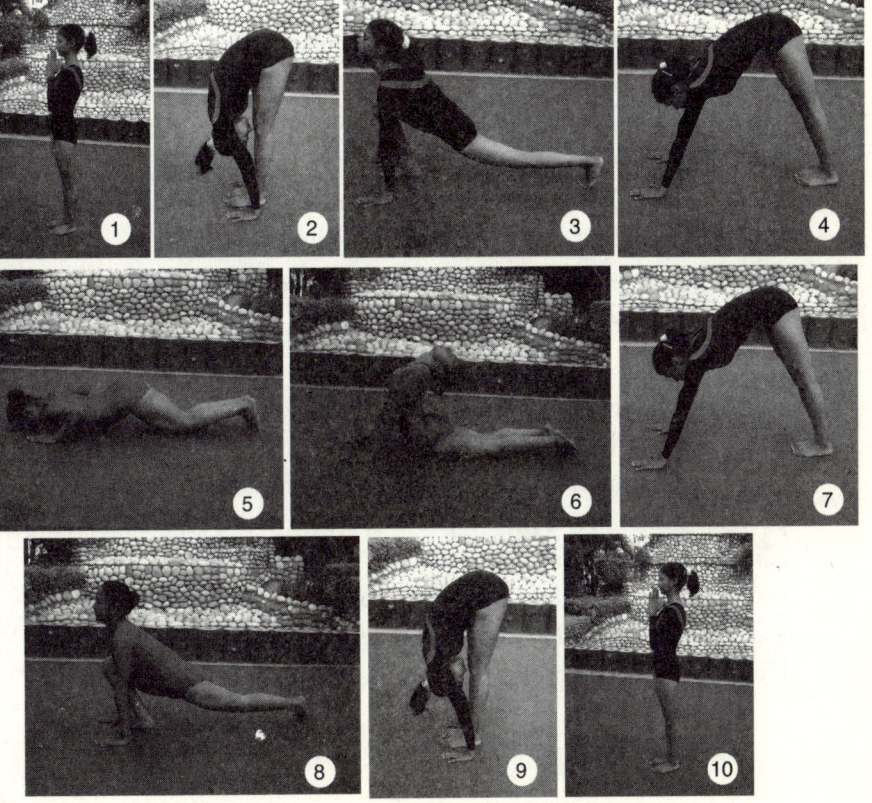

It invigorates the facial tissues, the central nervous system and the organs of the upper portion of the body.

- *Position 1*: Stand straight with hands folded.
- *Position 2*: Inhale slowly and bend forward raising both arms forward touching the floor or the feet.
- *Position 3*: Hold the breath for a while putting both hands on the floor. Raise the head stretching the left leg backward.
- *Position 4*: Now move the right leg also backwards to join the left foot.
- *Position 5*: Lower the chest resting the knees on the floor and chin also touching the floor.
- *Position 6*: Raise your head and chest off the floor. Bend your upper body as far back as you can keeping the arms straight.
- *Position 7*: Take a deep breath, and while exhaling, come back to the position of the fourth step, i.e. head towards the ground though not touching it, palms and feet on the ground and abdomen raised above the ground.
- *Position 8*: Bring the right leg forward and bend it at the knee. This position is same as in the third step.
- *Position 9*: As you inhale, bring the left leg also forward.
- *Position 10*: Return to the original starting position with folded hands.

Once the lochia has stopped, a breastfeeding mother may not have periods for several months after the childbirth. The breastfeeding mothers often have painful contractions. Post-birth pains are common and they stop after few days. If there is continuous pain or bleeding, consult your doctor. Constipation too, can be a problem if you have stitches. Do not push or strain while in toilet. Take care if you suffer from backache after the childbirth. Avoid lifting heavy weight during this period.

Massage for Painless Labour

Massage is a very important natural tool for painless delivery. Effleurage is a light, rhythmic, stroking massage of the abdomen, back and thighs to relieve pain during delivery. Some women prefer an extremely light, even 'tickly' stroking, while others find a firmer touch more soothing. Practise effleurage massage as part of your labour preparation during pregnancy. Effleurage over the lower abdomen in circles with both hands, following the lower curve of the uterus is most popular.

Many women use effleurage movements during contractions in labour. Keep the massage rhythmic, even timing it with slow breathing. If you find that your skin is becoming extra sensitive as the contractions intensify, try effleurage in a different area or discontinue it. Other type of massage movements, such as firm stroking or kneading are soothing and relaxing both during pregnancy and labour.

Another helpful massage movement for labour is known as counter-pressure, used particularly over the lower back during contractions. The person giving massage presses with fist or the heel of the hand on a spot in the lower back or on the side of the hips. The exact spot for applying pressure varies from woman to woman and changes during labour. It should be tried over various places to find out the most helpful spot.

Perineal massage during pregnancy has a different purpose than most massages. It is used to soften the tissues around the vagina and increase the elasticity of the perineum by taking advantage of the hormonal changes that loosen the connective tissues in late pregnancy. It also helps to relax the pelvic floor muscles affected by pressure from the enlarged uterus and during childbirth. Perineal massage can help avoid an episiotomy (a small cut). It is also helpful in quicker delivery and prevents undue downward pressure on the uterus and the adjoining parts like bladder and rectum.

To avoid an episiotomy, a pregnant woman may find it very helpful to massage the perineum daily for about six weeks before the expected due date of the delivery. If suffering from vaginitis, herpes or other vaginal problems avoid a perineal massage as it could worsen the condition. To give a perineal self-massage the following steps are taken:

- The first few times, take a mirror and look at your perineum to assess the procedure for giving massage.
- Be sure your fingernails are short.
- If you have a rough skin, wear disposable rubber gloves.
- Wash your hands before beginning the massage.
- Make yourself comfortable in a semi-sitting position, squatting against a wall, sitting on the toilet seat or standing with one foot up on a chair.
- Lubricate your fingers well with oil or water-soluble jelly. Some naturopaths recommend use of wheat germ oil, which contains high vitamin E contents. Vegetable oils or water-based lubricants such as K-Y jelly can also be used. Never use mineral oil or petroleum jelly. Wash your hands before dipping into the lubricant every time.
- Rub enough oil or jelly into the perineum to allow your fingers to move smoothly over the tissue and the lower vaginal wall.
- Use your thumb and index finger when doing self-massage. Put the index finger and the thumb well inside the vagina up to the second knuckle, move upward along the sides of the vagina in a rhythmic U or sling type movement. This movement will stretch the vaginal tissues, the muscles surrounding the vagina and the skin of the perineum.
- Concentrate on relaxing your muscles as you apply pressure. After regular practice increase the pressure just enough to enable a stinging sensation that occurs as the baby's head comes out at the time of delivery.
- Continue the massage for five minutes.

Recommended yogic exercises such as *dandymana janusirasana, janusir merudandasana, viparitakarniasana, nauli mudra, mulabandhasana* and *matsyasana* help in painless delivery.

Uterine Rupture

Breach of the uterine wall results in significant maternal or foetal morbidity or mortality. Rupture of an intact uterus does not occur in rare occasion. In most cases it prevails in women with a previous cesarean delivery or for whom vaginal birth after cesarean delivery fails. The main causes of a uterine rupture are the following:

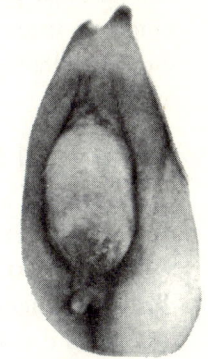

Ruptured Uterus

- Abnormal healing of the previous uterine scar.
- Mechanical disruption of the uterine wall weakened by previous surgery.
- Congenital anomalies or abnormalities of the placenta.
- Traumatic rupture of the uterus.
- Effect of an accident, which results in injury to both mother and foetus.

  Signs and symptoms of uterine rupture include:
- Abrupt foetal distress
- Vaginal bleeding
- Abdominal pain
- Maternal circulatory collapse
- Uterine dehiscence
- Placental abruption
- Umbilical cord prolapse

  An immediate operative delivery is required as a measure.

Uterine Postpartum

Loss of uterine tone after delivery that often presents a postpartum haemorrhage generally seen in about 5% cases is caused due to the loss of the normal uterine contractile forces. The risk factors include prolonged labour, prolonged oxytocin stimulation, uterine rupture, genital-tract laceration and retained placental tissue in the uterus.

Signs and symptoms of this disorder include bright red vaginal bleeding, loss of uterine tone palpable on the abdominal examination and vascular collapse. To treat this disorder massage the uterus fundus (portion above the uterus outside the body) and the bladder should be drained to allow the uterus to contract and to assess urinary output.

Leakage of Milk

Breasts are felt hard, sore and soaked because of the secretion of milk from them in early or mid-pregnancy often in the morning. Consult a gynaecologist who will teach you how to take care of the breasts during pregnancy. Give a firm support to the breasts using a good quality and correct-sized brassière, which should be loose and supportive, but not tight. Light exercises for the breasts should be done. Regular practice of *bhujangasana* and *dhanurasana* help a lot.

PROBLEMS OF PREGNANT WOMEN

Problem	*Cause*	*Recommended Yogic Cure*
Blood stained discharge	Generally, due to infection or erosion of the cervix. It is an alarming sign of problem pregnancy.	Have complete bed rest and consult a doctor immediately. Avoid yoga exercises.
Toxaemia of Pregnancy	The disease is characterised by body swelling, rise in blood pressure, breathlessness and excessive protein in the urine. Its cause is unknown.	Recommended yogic postures are — *Tarasana, vajrasana* and *shavasana.*
Vulvitis	Cause by infection, allergic reaction and ageing.	Avoid spices and condiments. A warm water douche should be given and a solution of camphor mixed with rose water should be applied inside the genital tract. Recommended yogic postures — *gomukhasana, ek pada uttanasana* and *yog mudra.*

Table contd...

Problem	Cause	Recommended Yogic Cure
Retention of urine	A common problem during the third trimester of pregnancy due to the weight of the foetus on the urethra.	Avoid strong diuretics. Recommended yogic postures: *supta vajrasana* and *ardha matsyendrasana.*
Hydramnios	Develops in women during 5th or 6th month of pregnancy and may result in miscarriage.	Avoid yoga exercises as far as possible.
Itching pain in vagina	Common disorder in women having regular secretion.	Avoid sex during pregnancy. Recommended yogic postures are – *yog mudra, malasana, supta vajrasana* and *pasasana.*
Pain in the lower abdomen	Due to weakness in pregnant women or infection in pelvic organs.	Recommended yogic postures are – *yog mudra* and *ardha chandrasana.*
Anaemia	A pregnant woman enters an anaemic condition usually in the 12th week due to the deficiency of blood and iron in the body and the condition reaches its climax in the 32nd week.	Recommended yogic postures are – *paschimottanasana, ardha matsyendrasana, shavasana* and regular practise of *pranayama.*
Breast inflammation	Hormonal imbalance	Recommended yogic postures are – *bhujangasana* and *dhanurasana.*
Displacement of the uterus	Occurs in late pregnancy when the uterus slips downwards in between the space of the bladder and bowel due to weight. It may produce offensive smell from the vagina due to infection.	Recommended yogic postures are – *gomukhasana, mandukasana* and *yog mudra.*

Table contd...

Problem	Cause	Recommended Yogic Cure
Heavy vaginal discharge	Usually due to local infection during pregnancy.	Recommended yogic postures are – *shallabhasana* and *ek pada uttanaasana*.
Morning sickness	Nausea usually in the morning during early stage of pregnancy or two week after conception.	Recommended yogic postures are – *Tarasana, virasana, uttanasana* and *marjarasana*.
Stomach or liver pain	Due to the increased weight of the embryo.	Massage the stomach gently with *ghee* to relieve pain and practise *pranayama*.
Cramps	The trouble starts during 4th month of pregnancy due to the deficiency of vitamins and minerals. The pain develops more in waist, stomach and muscles of the hips.	Massage the whole body with *narayani* oil. Recommended yogic postures are – *pasasana, mandukasana, garudasana* and *gomukhasana*.

3

Solution to the Common Sexual Problems

Decrease in Frequency of Sex

The frequency of sexual intercourse depends upon the couples suiting their moods and needs. The frequency of the sexual intercourse varies from couple to couple. Some need sex every day, others once or twice a month, even in their early years of marriage. With increase in age there is a decrease in the sexual desires and frequency of sex in most of the couples.

Recommended yogic exercises are – *paschimottanasana, mandukasana, sarvangasana, setubandha sarvangasana, supta vajrasana, viparita karniasana* and *janusirasana*

Contraceptive Methods

Various contraceptive methods for family planning have been described earlier. However, there are mainly three natural ways as below:

- *Coitus interruptus*: This is an unreliable and unhealthy method of contraception usually practised by traditional couples in which the sex act is interrupted at the time of male ejaculation and the male organ is quickly withdrawn out of the vagina before the semen is discharged. However, long-term practice of coitus interruptus can cause pelvic congestion with the formation of ovarian cysts in the female.

- *Rhythm method*: This method follows the natural ovulation pattern in women, which happens once a month on the 14th day of the cycle (immediately before and after this day are the most fertile days). However, the days following the menses and preceding the next period are the least fertile. The ovum is capable of getting fertilised for two or three days after its liberation. If the intercourse is avoided during ovulation and three to four days before and after, the chances of conception are minimal. It is very necessary to avoid having sex for over a week in the mid cycle. Men can also use a condom during this period.

- *Lactating the baby*: In many women, during total lactation, ovulation stops and menses do not take place. During this period a woman cannot conceive or has very low fertility. This method, too, is not hundred per cent reliable as there are instances, despite lactation, the woman conceives even before menstruation restarts. In some cases, menstruation and ovulation commence within three months of the delivery. The early restart of sex brings on quicker menstruation and ovulation due to hormonal effect on the system with decreasing breast milk.

Preventing Reproduction

Vasectomy

Sterilising the male or the female is the best way for preventing reproduction. In males the operation is called *vasectomy* in which the ducts (vas) carrying the sperms from the testes to the urethra in the penis is cut on both sides and tied beneath the skin of the scrotum. This operation is usually 100% successful. After getting vasectomy done there is no loss of libido, difficulty in performing the sex act or general debilitating effects. Vasectomy if performed unhygienically can produce infection in the internal genital organs. In few cases the operation causes minor nerve pain during erection.

Tubectomy

In females, the operation is known as *tubectomy* in which the fallopian tubes on either side are cut and ligatured. This operation is performed easily, even a week after the delivery of the child when the uterus is still high up in position and tubes are easy to ligature. The operation is performed by laparoscopy technique. A pencil like instrument fitted with microscope (micro surgery) is inserted through a small incision in the abdomen and the image is displayed on the TV-screen.

Infertility

Infertility, in human beings is the inability of a woman to conceive or of a man to father children. Both man and woman may be able to produce children with a different partner. Infertility in 60% of the cases is due to some problem in women. Causes of sterility in women:

- Defect in the sex organs
- Ovarian problems
- Hormonal disorders due to pituitary, thyroid or adrenal malfunction.
- Chemical anti-sperm action of the genital secretions.

Causes of sterility in men:

- Absence of sperms
- Low sperm count or a high percentage of sperm that do not function normally.
- Extremely frail sperms lose their mobility and vitality soon due to an auto immune reaction in the male's system that destroys his own sperms.

In some of the cases, women suffering from infertility are seen unable to conceive due to malfunctioning of the reproductive organs. In such cases females should take the treatment for anaemia and have a nutritious diet.

Here are a few naturopathic remedies to treat infertility among females:

- Ivory powder taken with milk for 3-4 days after the monthly periods cures this disorder.
- Tender aerial dried finely powdered roots of the banyan tree mixed with milk and taken before sleep for three days cures this disorder.

- Excessive fat often inhibits conception. In such cases obesity must be treated first. Yogic exercises to fight obesity are helpful in this case.

- A woman under treatment should avoid taking alkaline and pungent foods.

  Recommended yogic postures are — *yog mudra, shirshasana, salambha shirshasana, baddha konasana* and *mandukasana.*

Premature Ejaculation

It is a malfunctioning due to psychological reasons generally found in males who are sexually more aroused than the females, who need a bit of foreplay to be ready for the intercourse. Excessive indulgence in sexual fantasies and too much of excitement can lead to premature ejaculation, giving a feeling of failure or lack of fulfilment after the sexual intercourse. The following are the natural ways to treat premature ejaculation:

- Apply mud pack on the pubes before sleeping at night.

- Kegal Exercise: Squeeze the muscles in the anal area as if you are trying to stop the flow of urine. This exercise strengthens the pubococcygeus muscle, the urethra (urinary tube) and the rectum. A regular practice will help control premature ejaculation.

- Self-stimulation: Another way to treat premature ejaculation is self-stimulation. Masturbate three to four times a week, just bringing yourself close to orgasm but without ejaculating.

- Scrotal Pull Technique: During self-stimulation try to pull down on your scrotal sac before you reach the point of no return. During sex, you can do it yourself or seek the help of your partner.

- Press the area on your perineum, the space between the anus and the back of the scrotum, which stimulates the prostate – the gland that supplies the fluid for semen during ejaculation. Pressing on this spot when you are highly aroused helps block the ejaculatory reflex and can be quite pleasurable and delays ejaculation. Press on it firmly and rhythmically at any point on the area during sex after you have achieved a maximum erection.

- Mix equal quantities of *lajwanti* seeds and sugar and take it with the milk in the morning.
- Avoid constipation and stomach disorders.

Recommended yogic exercises are – *yog mudra, sarvangasana, viparitakarniasana, paschimottanasana, shirshasana, salambha shirshasana* and *baddha konasana.*

Impotence

Impotence (sexual weakness) is the inability to perform sex – it may be partial or complete, temporary or permanent. Impotence can result due to two reasons – organic or psychological, as described below:

Organic Impotence

It is caused by the following reasons:

- Lesions of the external genitalia such as a tight foreskin.
- Disturbances of the endocrine glands, such as diminished activity of the gonads, thyroid glands or pituitary glands.
- Diseases of the central nervous system.
- Severe disturbance of health.
- Diabetes

Psychological Impotence

It is caused by the following factors:

- Ignorance about sex
- Fear
- Weakness or abnormality of sexual desire.

The psychological treatment of impotence is to find the true reason that has caused it.

Treatment for Impotence

- The best remedy for impotence is a healthy diet and exercise.
- A wet pack (dipped in cold water) on the spine can help the body to energise and strengthen the nervous system. Lie naked on the bed so that the wet bandage remains in constant touch with the spine.

- Drink plenty of water in a day to wash away all the morbid matter that has been poisoning the body system.
- Dry in the shade tender and seedless pods of acacia and mix them with equal quantity of brown sugar. Take this mixture with milk. Alternatively, tender leaf-shoots of banyan tree may be substituted for acacia pods.

Recommended yogic postures are – *mandukasana, shirshasana, salambha shirshasana, viparitakarniasana* and *sarvangasana, halasana and paschimottanasana.*

Frigidity

Frigidity is a condition in a woman, where she is unable to give herself sexually to the male partner and enjoy sex usually due to the following reasons:

- Psychological fear.
- Wrong notions about sex.
- Physical incapacity.
- Hormonal and genital defects.
- Cultural taboos and social position.
- Intellectual upbringing and emotional status playing a significant role in a female's sexual behaviour.
- Sexual indifferences (which is the major reason) or disliking for sex.
- Physical causes such as inflamed vagina, a very rigid hymen, urinary problems or uterine infections.
- Displaced ovaries.

Recommended yogic exercises are – *yog mudra, mandukasana* and *viparitakarniasana.*

Male Sterility

This disorder also recognised as sexual weakness is the failure to fertilise the ovum or the female egg cells due to the following reasons:

- Some obstruction in the male genital organs.
- Infection involving male genital organs.

- Production of weak and dead sperm cells.
- Lack of normal sex desire, rather than any deficiency of hormones.
- Emotional factors such as anxiety and worry, which may bring on the feelings of guilt and weakness.

Male sterility may be cured by the following ways:
- Take 50 mg of vitamin E tablets thrice a day.
- Take a healthy diet full of vitamins.
- In case the disorder is due to psychological reasons, consult a psychiatrist.

Nocturnal Emission

Involuntary discharge of semen (the fluid produced by the testicles in male) during sleep or nocturnal emission is one of the common disorders among youths and even in middle-age people. Night emission among youngsters is generally due to excitement because of reading vulgar literature or seeing sexually explicit scenes on television. The following treatments are recommended to cure this psychological disorder:
- Avoid thoughts of sex.
- Eat rich food.
- Have dinner three hours before sleep.
- Go for evening walk followed by a bath.
- Go to bed early, not late than 9 p.m.
- Apply mud pack on the pubes during sleep at night.
- Hot and cold hip bath.

    Recommended yogic exercises are – *baddha konasana, mula-bandha, yog mudra* and *virbhadrasana.*

Painful Intercourse

The disorder is also known as dyspareunia, which may arise from muscular spasm of the vagina. Sometimes, there is a superficial ulceration following some injury. Bladder infection is common in such cases, which may lead to further complications.

Some of the causes of a painful intercourse are:

- Tightness in the female genital area after a surgery. In such case usually tissues may have been drawn too tightly together.
- Pelvic inflammation may cause pain during intercourse.
- Nervous tension usually due to being unconsciously afraid of pregnancy.
- Problems like body odours, halitosis, etc.
- Lack of understanding on the part of the male partner.

Recommended yogic exercises are – *baddha konasana, yog mudra, malasana* and *pasasana.*

Honeymoon Urethritis

Over enthusiastic love-making, excessive handling of the clitoris during foreplay, having intercourse too frequently after the marriage leads to severe inflammation of the urethral opening resulting in honeymoon urethritis. If the vagina has got infected or the infection is severe, pus cells pass into the bladder and higher up. In such a case, consult a doctor for immediate treatment.

Phosphaturia (Whitish discharge)

A whitish liquid discharged with urine in both sexes is called phosphaturia, i.e. the emission of phosphates. Usually this disorder is caused by indigestion. Fasting for a couple of days or consuming only fruits can clear the problem. Consult a doctor in case you feel weak after urinating. Go for a urine test.

Quite often lesions of scabies may be seen on the male genitals with intense itching. These lesions are observed as papules on the prepuce, glans, shaft of penis and scrotum with burrow tract on top in male organs.

4

Venereal Diseases

Syphilis

It is one of the greatest scourges ever to hit the human race. It is a dangerous venereal disease caused by a little corkscrew-shaped germ. This tiny germ is transmitted from one person to another mainly through sexual contact. In a few cases syphilis is acquired through contaminated materials and even through injections or blood transfusion, if the germs are present in the blood. If a mother is infected with syphilis, the germs may find their way into the child's body before birth.

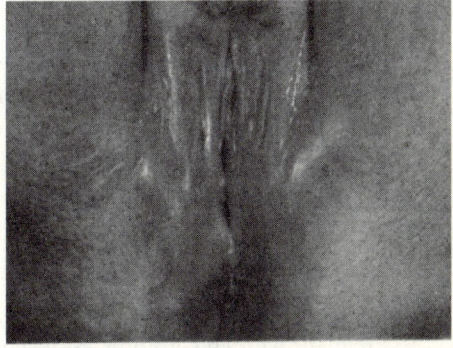

Advanced stage

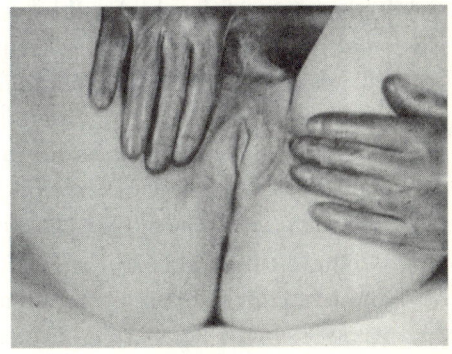

Initial stage

Signs and Symptoms

In males there may be a painless sore on the penis lasting several weeks. In females there may be a deep sore in the vagina. This early primary lesion is known as a chancre. At first the germs are generally confined to these areas, and later they are carried to all parts of the body through the blood and spread all over, causing mild rashes on the skin that fade in a short time. This is the secondary stage of the disease.

In the late stage tumours or swellings may appear in various parts of the body and there may be severe inflammation and degeneration. The nervous system is often affected with disastrous results involving the brain and the spinal cord resulting in headaches, loss of memory, tremors of the lips, tongue, fingers, hands and changes in the pupils of the eyes. In this disease the syphilis germ attacks the nerve roots coming from the spinal cord. There may be vomiting and acute abdominal pain lasting for hours or even days. Large ulcers may develop on the toes, heels, and soles, and there is often a loss of normal bladder control in the late stage of the disease. In some cases a large swelling may develop under the skin in several places including the inner organs of the body such as the stomach and liver. There may also be a loss of vision.

Pregnant women suffering from syphilis may pass on the disease to their unborn child resulting in serious conditions. Soon after the birth, the bones of the child will appear somewhat deformed, the liver and spleen enlarged. There may be damage to the brain and central nervous system causing a child to be retarded both mentally and physically. Besides, syphilitic mothers run the greatest risk of recurrent abortions and stillbirths due to the infection and damage to the placenta and the growing embryo. The following naturopathic remedies are recommended to treat syphilis:

- Ground a tablespoon of *Hirankhuri booti* (corchorus fascicularis) and five grains of pepper. Strain and take it for two to three weeks.
- Take a salt-free diet. Avoid taking bitter, sour and pungent foods.

Recommended yogic exercises are *bhunamanasana, kurmasana, upavista konasana, adho mukha shavanasana, supta vajrasana, ushtrasana, viparitakarniasana* and *dhanurasana*.

Upavistha Konasana (wide leg forward bend)

In this asana sit on the ground spreading legs in front. Widen the legs sideways one by one and tighten the leg muscles. Also try to hold your ankles with both hands. Bend forward resting the forehead or chin on the floor. Rotate waist to right and hold right foot with both hands resting forehead or chin on the knee. Return to the initial position, rotate the waist to left, hold left feet and repeat the exercise.

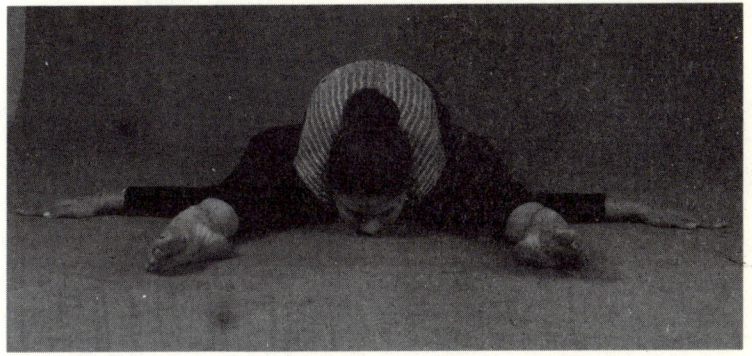

Upavistha Konasana

Benefits

This yogic posture improves circulation in the pelvic region, makes the hamstring muscles elastic and strengthens the muscles of the spinal column.

Adho Mukha Shavanasana

Adho means 'down', *Mukha* means 'face' and *Shavana* means 'dog'. To practise this posture stand straight. Bend forward and rest your palms on the floor in front. Keep your feet about 12 inches apart. Lift your hips up and tighten the thighs stretching like a dog to form an inverted 'V'. Rest the head on the floor.

Gonorrhoea

Persistent pus discharge from the vagina, inflammation of the entire genital passage, burning and discomfort – all these symptoms indicate the presence of a fatal venereal disease – gonorrhoea. It is a venereal disease, which is almost always transmitted by sexual contact caused by a tiny bean-shaped germ called 'gonococcus'. In some cases, the disease may also be contracted from contaminated

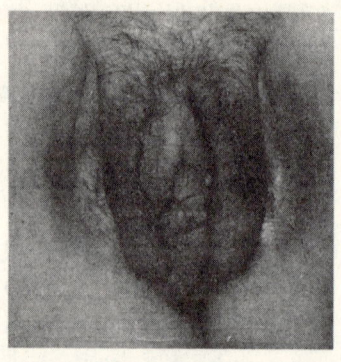

Gonorrhoea

hands, instruments, clothing and toilet seats.

The symptoms are as following:

- Burning sensation during urination.
- Urge for frequent urination (cystitis).
- A profuse, greenish-yellow discharge.
- In males the tip of the penis may be red and swollen.
- In females, the glands around the opening of the vagina may be hot and swollen, and there may be thick yellow discharge during the acute initial stage.

Many adult women carry gonorrhoea germs for a long period of time and may readily transmit the germs during sexual intercourse. If a mother happens to be infected with gonorrhoea, there is a great danger of the newborn infant contracting the disease at the time of birth. Unless the infant is properly treated, he may become completely blind later in life. Sometimes, sterility results from this serious infection in females. In the males the prostate gland becomes infected resulting in slow urination. In females, the fallopian tubes get closed and abscesses and inflammation may spread to the whole pelvis. The following treatments cure gonorrhoea:

- Penicillin or terramycin are the best drugs for treating this fatal disease under the guidance of an expert doctor as there may be a reaction due to these drugs.

- Hip bath in hot water is useful.
- Urethra should be flushed with a solution of potassium permanganate (1:3000). The solution should be kept in the urethra for five minutes with the help of a syringe.
- Avoid constipation. It should be dealt with a mild laxative.
- Sex should be strictly forbidden during the period of the disorder.

Recommended yogic postures are – *kurmasana, bhunamanasana* and *supta vajrasana, matsyasana.*

Genital Herpes

Genital herpes is a common sexually transmitted disease caused by herpes simplex virus type 2 and is passed on through sexual contact. First infection with genital herpes can show up as blisters on the skin usually on the genitals, thighs and buttocks. Other symptoms include fever, bodyache, weakness, vaginal discharge and irritation, urinary burning and enlarged lymph nodes. Different sized vesicles and reddish ulcers are noticed in the vulva region. The subsequent attacks may be confined to few blebs and ulcers in the vaginal mucous membrane. Women who practise rectal sex develop the lesions in the area around the anus and higher up in the rectum. This disease is controlled by the following treatments:

- Apply anti-viral cream or a lotion.
- Use condoms during sexual intercourse.
- Take bath in warm water.
- Leave apart worry, depression and take proper sleep.
- Soothe the affected skin with essential oil (diluted in a base oil) of lemon, geranium, chamomile or lavender. The oil should be rubbed on to the rash.

Recommended yogic postures are – *yog mudra* and *sarvangasana.*

Natural Remedies to Cure Genital Herpes

- A herpes outbreak is a sign that your body is under stress and whenever you are under stress you need more nutrients.

- Drink as much water as you can, which helps in flushing out toxins that weaken your immune system allowing the virus to reactivate.
- The group of little blisters appearing on the genital area can be cured by applying essential oils (diluted in a base oil) of lemon, geranium, chamomile or lavender.
- Common warts are treated by electro-cautery, which excises the warts with electric current.

The following nutrient programme may help reduce the stress, thus reducing the severity of a herpes attack.

Vitamin A	: Daily dose of 20,000 international units (IU) twice for a week.
Vitamin B Complex	: Daily dose of 50mg for a month.
Vitamin C	: Daily dose of 500 to 1000 mg three times for one to two weeks.
Vitamin E	: 400 IU twice a day for two weeks.
Zinc	: 10mg twice a day for a week.
Calcium/Magnesium	: 500mg of calcium and 250mg of magnesium twice a day for a month.
Selenium	: 200 micrograms daily for two weeks.

HIV and AIDS

Aids virus depresses immunity, increases the risk of common and rare infections and rare cancers. HIV (human immunodeficiency virus) is the virus that causes AIDS – disease that destroys the immune system and ravages the body. It may be transmitted heterosexually or by infected blood transfusion. Use of condoms reduces the risk. It is primarily confined to male homosexuals, addicts used to intravenous drug abuse, those receiving blood transfusion or other blood products. The virus can be sexually transmitted from man to man, man to woman, woman to man and infected mother to her child. Heterosexual transmission in promiscuous individuals has been observed with frequent exchange of partners. So far there is no effective treatment for AIDS. Fever, loss of weight, recurrent diarrhoea, extreme fatigue, glandular enlargement, severe toxicity and lack of resistance to fight infection, tumours and pneumonia bring the end. Certain degree of sexual restrain with a healthy, happy monogamous relationship is the only answer to stop the spread of the disease.

There is no cure for AIDS, no ways to eradicate HIV from the body. Infections and other skin problems are common in people with HIV. There is need of sufficient protein by a patient suffering from this dreaded disease. For vegetarians a daily supplement containing 4,000 to 6,000 mg of flaxseed oil is recommended. For non-vegetarians, a daily supplement of both fish oil in 2,000 to 4,000 mg doses and borage oil in 240 to 480 mg doses may be helpful. Garlic, contains allicin, a powerful compound that can help kill bacteria, fungi and viruses. An HIV patient should take at least 9 gm of raw garlic a day in the form of juice or three medium cloves. Garlic can be taken in three doses of 3 gm each at morning, noon and evening. The garlic juice can be added to fresh juices.

Genital Warts

Genital warts can occur in both sexes and are usually located on the moist surface of genitalia and appear as minute reddish swelling growing in groups of lesions. Genital warts are usually transmitted by sexual contact or through infection from the hands. Both the partners should keep their hands clean when having sex. The genital warts should be treated with the consultation of a good doctor. Apply recommended cream or lotion on the affected organs and its surrounding area should be protected with petroleum jelly. Painful, tender, highly infectious genital herpes are caused by virus. It is more common among youngsters. Groups of little blisters appear on the genital area, thighs and buttocks.

Warts should be diagnosed accurately and treated appropriately. It is important to treat them early rather than waiting until they spread and enlarge and are more difficult to eliminate. Genital warts can be sexually transmitted and may be a risk factor for cervical cancer in women.

To treat warts following remedies are advised:

- Garlic oil is a traditional remedy for warts. Swab the oil on the wart or on a bandage which then should be put on the wart.

- If the wart is soft, fleshy, bleeds easily, then apply the homoeopathic medicine *'Thuja Occidentalis'* (in 30X potency). You may consult a homoeopath for proper dose.

- Remove warts with cryosurgery or freeze them with liquid nitrogen or carbon snow.

Scabies

Scabies is a contagious disease caused by a mite, which lays eggs in the burrows in the skin. The disease spreads through contact with an infected individual. The commonly affected parts of the body are finger webs, wrists, arms, buttocks, lower abdomen, thighs, breast-folds, female genital area and penis (in men). There is severe itching on the affected area at night and sometimes a thin, slimy fluid oozes out of the scratched surface and scabs. To treat scabies following remedies are advised:

- Boil the leaves of oleander (*karbir*) till charred in 250 ml mustard oil and massage the affected skin with this.

- Mix the juices of lemon and jasmine in equal quantities and rub on the itching skin.

- Grind poppy seeds in water and add lime juice to it. Massage the affected area with the paste.

5

Female Genital Diseases

DISEASES OF VULVA

Bartholin's Glands

It is a vulva disease, causing abscesses or cysts due to infection, resulting in swelling and/or formation of abscess. The pain occurs during the reproductive years of the female. The signs and symptoms include:

- Painful swelling of the labia on vulva.
- Masonephric cysts on the vagina.
- Sebaceous cysts.
- Yellow or blue colour smooth and smaller cysts are seen at the base of the labia majora.

To prevent the disease, avoid or refrain from unprotected sex.

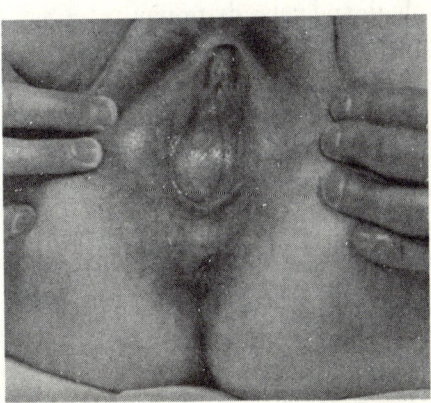

Contact Vulvitis

Vulva irritation is caused by contact with an irritant as a result of the following factors:

- Unhygienic conditions
- Effect of using deodorants, scented soaps and perfumes on the genital area.
- Wearing tight-fitting and synthetic undergarments, tampons or pads.
- Using condoms, lubricants, topical contraceptives and sexual aids.
- When semen remains in the vagina.
- Soiling of vulva by urine or faeces.

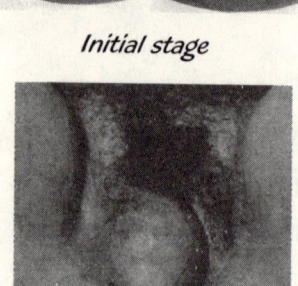

Initial stage

Advanced stage

The signs and symptoms of this disorder include:

- Severe dermatitis of the vulva.
- Reddening of the vulva skin accompanied by itching and burning.
- Atrophic vulvitis and vulva dystrophy.
- Ailments such as pinworms, psoriasis, seborrheic dermatitis, neurodermatitis, impetigo and vaginal secretions.

Dyspareuria Insertional

It is pain or discomfort in the vaginal or pelvic area experienced by a woman during sexual intercourse. This pain may lead to severe vaginal spasm that interferes with penetration.

The signs and symptoms include:

- Burning or pinching sensation of the vulva, perineum and the outer portion of the vagina.

- The disease is common among women during the reproductive age. It is generally caused due to congenital factors, insufficient foreplay, inadequate lubrication, phobias about sex, pelvic muscle spasm, scarring due to episiotomy, surgical repairs of the vulva, vulvitis, urethral syndrome, urethritis and herpes vulvitis.

Treatment includes the following:

- Vaginal lubrication.
- Regular practice of pelvic relaxation exercises.
- Sexual techniques to reduce pain during intercourse.
- Improved position during sexual intercourse.

Female Circumcision

Female circumcision is removing the part or external genital organs, including labia majora, labia minora and clitoris.

The signs and symptoms of this disorder are following:

- Scarring and deformity of the external genitalia structures.
- Obstruction causing menstrual disorders such as amenorrhoea or dysmenorrhoea.
- Orgasmic dysfunction (dyspareunia).
- Burn injuries, inter-sex conditions and imperforate hymen.
- Possible complications include bleeding, infection, urinary retention, pain and sexual dysfunction.
- Urinary-tract infections, defective menstruation and pelvic inflammatory diseases.

Treatment includes the following:

- Surgical opening of fused/scarred genital tissues.
- Menstruation hygiene.
- Episiotomy required at the time of childbirth.

Hidradenitis Suppurativa

A chronic refractory infection of the skin and subcutaneous tissues causing inflammation of aprocrine glands and formation of abscess involving vulva and perineum.

Hidradenitis suppurativa usually occurs as multiple lumps that are firm and tender. They vary in size from 1cm to 3 cm (occasionally larger) and may open and drain pus.

The signs and symptoms include:

• Recurrent inflammation of the labia with severe pain.

• Foul smelling discharge.

• Formation of abscess.

• sexually transmitted diseases.

General measures for the treatment of this disease are the following:

• Perineal hygiene.

• Sitz's bath.

• Administering antibiotics and topical steroids in consultation with a doctor.

• Oral contraceptives and use of anti-androgens.

• Preventing the formation of scarring, abscesses, infection and sexual dysfunction.

Hymenal Stenosis

Thickening or narrowing of the opening of the hymen, resulting in difficulty in intercourse caused by congenital narrowing of the hymen or scarring after surgery or trauma. It can be diagnosed by vulva vestibulatis, vaginismus and vulvitis. Evaluation, gentle digital dilation and surgical excision are general measures to treat this disease. If not treated timely, it may cause complication of sexual dysfunction.

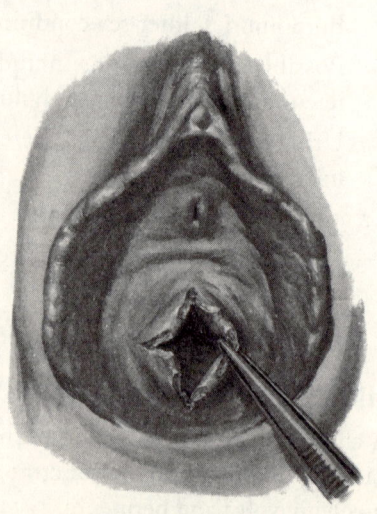

Hymenal Stenosis

Vulva Dystrophy

Vulva Dystrophy is the thickening of the vulva skin over the labia majora, labia minora and clitorial areas with inflammation and irritation. The signs and symptoms of this disease include:

- Itching of the vulva.
- White appearance of vulva.
- Fissuring and excoriations of the vulva.
- If not treated timely, the disease can cause cancer of the vulva, chronic vulvitis, psoriasis, vulvar pruritis and dyspareunia.

To treat this disease the following measures are adopted:

- Perineal hygiene.
- Stress reduction.
- Sitz's bath.
- Reducing candidiasis or contact allergy.

The patient should strictly take the following precautions:

- Wear gloves during night to avoid tissue damage due to scratching.
- Use perineal soothing preparations to reduce itching.
- If not treated well in time, the patient may suffer from cancer of the vulva.

Imperforated Hymen

It may result from abnormalities in the development of canalisation of ducts resulting in vaginal obstructions, mild bleeding (amenorrhoea) and abdominal pain, which can be diagnosed by ultrasonography of the upper genital tract. This disorder can be treated by incision of the hymen and drainage of the vaginal canal. If not treated timely, it may lead to serious complications like scarring and narrowing of the hymen after surgical incision.

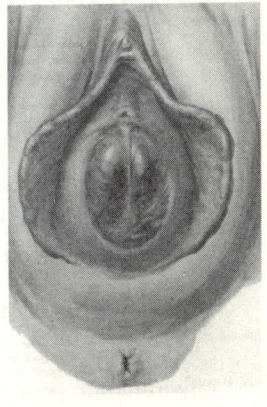

Imperforated Hymen

Labial Adhesions

It may be caused by local inflammation resulting in labial infections or irritation. This disorder consists of the following symptoms:

- Fusion of labia majora just below the clitoris.
- Retention of the urine resulting in irritation, discharge and odour.
- Female circumcision.
- Sexual abuse.
- Urinary-tract infection and vaginal bleeding.

Following measures are adopted to treat this disorder:

- Perineal hygiene.
- Sitz's bath.
- Use of topical estrogen cream.
- If not treated timely, complications like vaginitis and vaginal cyst may arise.

Lichen Planus

This disorder consists of the following symptoms:

- Red erosion.
- Ulceration of vulva.
- Oral lesion in labia minora and post-coital bleeding.

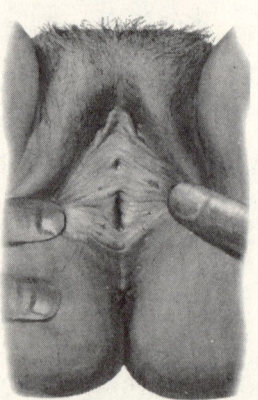

  To treat the disease, measures like local cleansing and surgical treatment are adopted. It would be better to consult a doctor. If not treated timely, there is a possibility of formation of the vulva lesion.

Lichen Planus

Lichen Sclerosus

Lichen Sclerosus is a chronic condition of the skin causing inflammation generally during late reproductive to early menopausal age.

The disease causes intense itching, scratch marks or fissures around the anus. It may result in hyper-plastic vulva dystrophy, Preget's disease, vulva candidiasis and carcinoma. The following measures are adopted to treat this disorder:

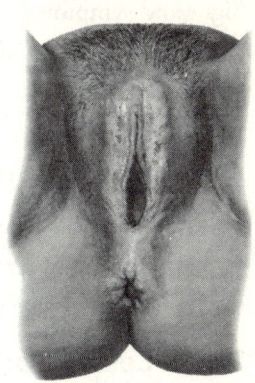

- Perineal hygiene.
- Sitz's bath and applying moist soaks.
- Wearing loose-fitting clothes.
- Applying petroleum jelly.

If not treated timely, complications such as the cancer of the vulva, scarring and narrowing of the vaginal canal may arise.

Lichen Sclerosus

Vulva Cancer

Presence of ulcer and lesions mostly in the age group of 60 to 70 are seen in this disorder. Itching, irritation, cracking and bleeding of the vulva are the common signs and symptoms of this disease, which can be detected by biopsy of suspicious lesion on the vulva. Other ailments include carcinoma of the clitoris, carcinoma of leukoplakia and sarcoma of the labium.

Vulva Hematoma

This disease consists of swelling of one or both labia because of interstitial bleeding occurring at any age and caused by an injury, sexual abuse, subject to rape, water skiing, vaginal surgery, delivery of child, effect of varicose veins of the vulva and sports activities.

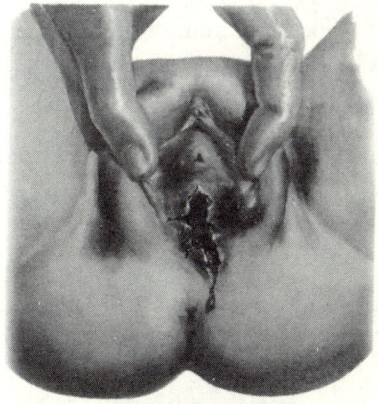

Vulva Hematoma

Signs and symptoms of this disorder include the following:
- Painful swelling of one or both labia.
- Dark blue or black discolouration of the vulva.
- Bleeding from the vulva.
- Formation of cysts, abscesses and varicose veins on the vulva.

Following are the measures to treat this disease:
- Application of ice packs.
- Surgical drainage in case of rapidly expanding symptoms.

Vulva Lesions and Cysts

The skin of vulva varies as similar to the skin elsewhere in the body. The tissues of the vulva have close interactions with the fluids, hormones and microbes in the body. The skin of the vulva like the skin of the other parts of the body contains hair follicles, sebaceous, sweat and apocrine glands, and is affected by inflammatory and various other skin diseases such as atopic dermatitis, psoriasis, seborrheic dermatitis, varicose veins, genitalia herpes, sebaceous cysts, senileatrophy, canal disorders, leukoplakia, vulvitis, parasitis, Bartholin's disease and viral infection.

The signs and symptoms of this disease include:
- Severe irritation.
- Vaginal secretions.
- Fleshy tumour of the vulva and recurrent urinary loss.
- The lesions and cysts, which appear on the vulva.

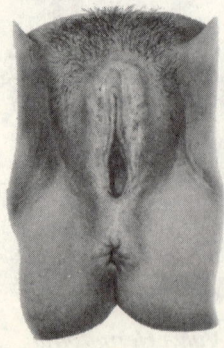

Senileatrophy

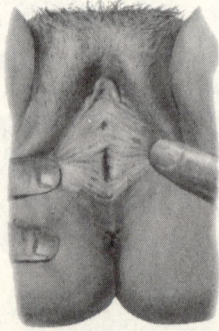

Kraurosis vulvae

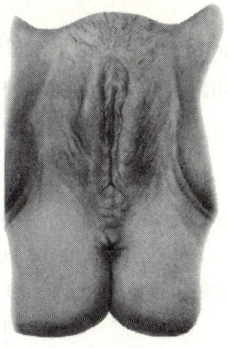

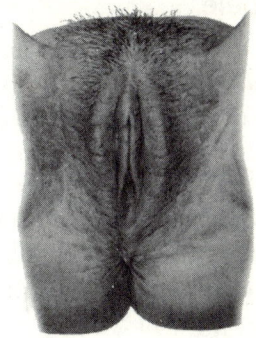

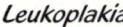
Leukoplakia   *Lichenification*

DISEASES OF THE VAGINA

Cystocele/Urethrocele

Following are the causes of these diseases:

- Lack of support due to ruptured vagina.
- Prolapse of the urethra (urethrocele) or bladder (cystocele) due to loss of normal tissue integrity caused by trauma such as childbirth, obstetric injury, surgery, etc.
- Pressure on the pelvic region.
- Urinary infections.
- Bulging of the tissues at the vaginal opening.
- Cysts, tumours and abscesses on the urethra.

The following measures are advised to treat this disorder:

- Weight-reduction.
- Treatment of cough, if present.
- Topical estrogen replacement therapy.
- Pelvic muscle exercises.
- Surgical repairs.
- Avoiding heavy lifting and straining.

Consult a doctor immediately in case of vaginal bleeding and symptoms of breast cancer.

Enterocele

It occurs due to the rupture or prolapse of the vaginal walls after abdominal or vaginal hysterectomy. Weight reduction and surgical repair are the main remedial measures.

Rectocele

Failure of the normal support mechanism between the rectum and the vagina as a result of childbirth, obstetric injury and surgery, obesity, heavy lifting and intrinsic tissue weakness cause this disorder.

The main signs and symptoms of this disease are the following:

- Bulging of the posterior vaginal wall.
- Difficulty in passing stool.
- Risk of a rectal cancer.
- Vaginal cyst after episiotomy (a cut on the opening of the vagina at the time of delivery of the child).
- Uterine prolapse.

The measures to treat this disorder are the following:

- Weight-loss.
- Treatment of chronic cough (if present).
- Systemic estrogen replacement.
- Pelvic muscle exercises.
- Surgical repair.

Sarcoma Botryoides

Tumour arising from the cervix are usually seen on the vagina of teenage girls, which causes vaginal bleeding and discharge of fleshy mass resembling a cluster of grapes. Other symptoms include urethral prolapse, vaginal polyp and indodermal sinus tumour. Surgical excision is the only treatment.

Vaginal Cysts

A vaginal cyst is a closed sac on or under the vaginal lining that contains fluid or semisolid material. Vaginal cysts are common in females from adolescence to middle reproductive years generally caused due to factors, e.g. episiotomy or obstetric laceration and gynaecological surgery. Vaginal cysts usually do not cause symptoms although there may be a soft lump felt in the vaginal wall or protruding from the vagina.

Cystic mass lesions ranging up to 5 cm are found in the lateral vaginal wall. Surgical excision is the only reliable treatment.

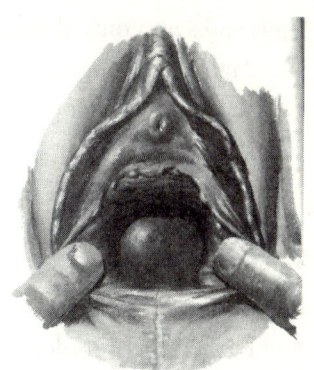

Vaginal Cysts

Vaginal Dryness

Loss of normal vaginal moisture results in irritation, itching or pain during sexual intercourse, inflamed vaginal tissue, vaginitis and vulva.

The causes of vaginal dryness are:

- Inadequate or inappropriate sexual stimulation.
- Sexual phobia.
- Pain more commonly after menopause.

Following are the measures to treat this disease.

- Topical moisturising and lubrication of the vagina.
- Estrogen replacement therapy.
- Counselling regarding sexuality.
- Foreplay.
- Use of water-soluble lubricants.

If not treated properly, it may lead to vaginal lacerations, infections, vulva excoriations and sexual dysfunction.

Vaginal Laceration

It is caused due to frequent sexual intercourse generally in the reproductive age, injury, sexual assault, penetration by foreign objects that cause, vaginismus, post-menopausal vaginal atrophy, hysterectomy and use of alcohol and drugs.

Signs and symptoms of this disorder include:

- Vaginal bleeding.
- Acute pain during intercourse and persistent pain after the intercourse.
- Cervical polyp.
- Excessive menstrual bleeding.
- Threatened abortion.

Following are the measures to treat this disease:

- To treat this disorder, have pelvic rest and avoid sex until healing occurs.
- Pack the vagina with sterilised guage in case of bleeding.

Vaginal Prolapse

It occurs due to the loss of normal support resulting in vaginal wall-down in the vaginal canal. In extreme cases vagina is displaced beyond the vulva outside the body. Childbirth, surgery, intra-abdominal pressure, chronic cough, heavy lifting, intrinsic tissue weakness and atrophic changes resulting from estrogen loss are some of the prominent causes of vaginal prolapse.

Signs and symptoms of this disorder include conditions such as:

- Urinary incontinence.
- Pelvic pain.
- Uterus dyspareunia.
- Inter-menstrual or post-menopausal bleeding
- Vaginal cyst or tumour.

The beneficial measures to treat this disorder are:

- Pessary therapy.
- Surgical and estrogen replacement therapy (Avoid estrogen therapy if undiagnosed vaginal bleeding exists).

Vaginitis Atrophic

Atrophy of the vaginal tissues is caused by the loss of ovarian steroids generally in post-menopausal women above the age of 50, and is usually caused as a result of surgery, chemotherapy, radiation or natural cessation of the ovarian function. The disease can be diagnosed by vaginal infection, hot flushes, sleep disturbance and vulvitis.

The signs and symptoms of the disease are as follows:

- Vaginal dryness.
- Burning and itching.
- Pain or bleeding during intercourse.
- Appearance of thin, shiny, red epithelium with a smooth surface.

Vaginal moisturiser and lubricants should be used during intercourse. Oral or injected estrogen treatment is also helpful.

Bacterial Vaginitis

Bacterial vaginitis is a vaginal infection caused by an over-growth of normal or pathogenic bacteria which causes severe itching, irritation and inflammation in the genital area between the age of 15 to 50. The causes of bacterial vaginitis are –

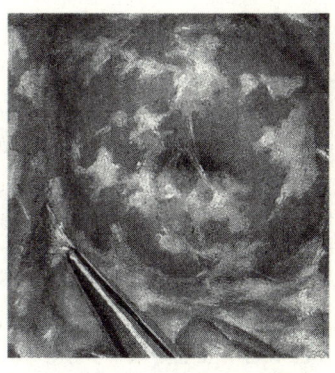

Bacterial Vaginitis

- Diabetes.
- Pregnancy and any debilitating disease.
- Excessive smoking.
- Multiple sexual partners.
- Excessive use of vaginal contraceptives.
- Oral sex.
- Unhygienic conditions.
- Menstruation and douche.

Perineal hygiene is an important measure to treat this disorder. If neglected, the possible complications like cystitis, cervicitis, severe infections, pelvic inflammatory disease, pelvic pain, infertility, increased risk of the upper genital-tract infection, premature delivery and premature rupturing of the membranes take place.

Vaginitis-monilial

Vaginitis-monilial is a vaginal infection caused by the ubiquitous fungi which are found in the atmosphere and are common inhabitants of the vagina, rectum and the vaginal mouth. It usually occurs in females between 15 to 50 years of age. Nearly 80 to 90 % cases of this disease are caused by candida albicus. The remaining cases are caused due to candida glabrata or candida tropicals.

The signs and symptoms of the disease are as follows:

- Vulva itching or burning and scratching.
- Oedema, vulva excoriations and white or yellow thick discharge.
- Bacterial vaginitis, vaginal infection, allergic vulvitis and pinworms.

Following are the important measures to treat the disease:

- Always keep the affected area clean and dry.
- Avoid wearing tight synthetic undergarments.
- Avoid topical steroid preparations.
- Avoid stress, diabetes, depression, topical contraceptives and warm and moist environments.

Vaginitis Trichomonas

Vaginitis trichomonas is a vaginal infection common in females between the age of 15 and 50 and is caused by the following reasons:

- Multiple sexual partners.
- Vaginal pH (less acid in blood and semen).

Signs and symptoms of this disease are the following:

- Vulva itching or burning.
- Watery yellow-green or gray colour discharge.
- Dysuria, dyspareunia and oedema of the vulva.
- Sexually transmissible infections.
- If not treated properly, it leads to complications like cystitis (inflammation of the bladder resulting in frequent urge to pass urine accompanied by pain in the lower abdomen), pelvic inflammation, infertility and pelvic pain.

The disorder can be cured by medical treatment. Consult a doctor immediately.

Candidiasis (White Vaginal Thrush)

Females during reproductive age sometimes suffer from candida. Factors like pregnancy, diabetes, administration of antibiotics and steroids and also the use of contraceptive pills cause this disorder. It produces white vaginal discharge with intense irritation and burning sensation on the affected area. The treatment consists of the application of anti-fungal preparations on the skin's surface to eliminate the

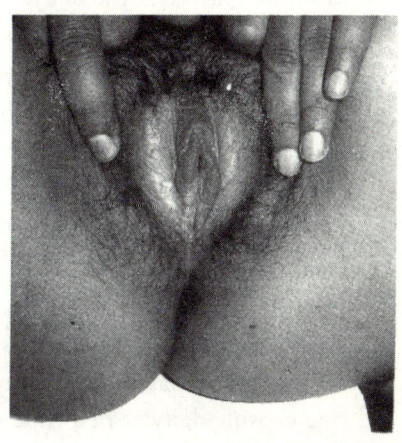

Candidiasis

fungus while preventing reinfection from the partner. Anti-fungal creams are generally recommended for both males and females. In females, doctors generally recommend tablets which are inserted intra-vaginally.

Thrush is another common infection. It is a disorder of candida which usually develops in the gastro-intestinal tract, in which whitish curd-like deposit appears on the tongue. The thrush infection of vagina is also known as vulva vaginitis, which causes itching, redness and discharge. The vaginal infection can be transmitted to the male partner and vice versa.

Symptoms of candida vaginitis include:

*   Pain, redness and itching in the vagina and vulva.
*   Severe pain while urinating.
*   Pain during sexual intercourse.
*   Foul smelling white or blood-streaked discharge.
*   Pelvic inflammation resulting in infertility.

Following are some of the naturopathic remedies for the treatment of candidiasis:

- *Sugar:* Avoid sugar, refined carbohydrates and alcohol, which turn into glucose in the body.

- *Yogurt:* Eat 100 gm of unsweetened yogurt with lactobacillus acidophilus bacteria daily for two weeks or take three capsules of a supplement of the bacterium between meals or use the capsules L. acidophilus as vaginal suppositories, inserting one capsule each morning for two weeks.

- *Garlic:* Garlic is antibacterial/ anti-fungal, which fights both bacterial vaginitis and candidiasis. Take one capsule once or twice a day.

- *Boric Acid:* Insert a 600 mg capsule of boric acid powder into the vagina twice a day for seven days. To prevent recurrence insert one capsule daily at bed time for four days during menstrual period. Do not insert capsule in case of pregnancy.

- *Vitamin E:* Use a gelatin capsule of vitamin E as a suppository, which is soothing to the vaginal tissue and decreases irritation, redness, swelling and congestion. Insert a capsule into the vagina once or twice a day for seven days.

- *Triphla:* Ayurvedic herb '*triphla*' helps remove toxins from the body; thus important in treating a yeast infection. Soak ½ teaspoon of dried herb in 1 cup of hot water for five minutes. Drink this liquid at night before sleep. Douche can also dry the vagina.

Note : Avoid wearing nylon panties and tight jeans.

Vaginal Infections

Yellow discharge from the vagina accompanied by itching can be due to fungal or bacterial infection. Candid V6/V3 is used for treating fungal infection. For bacterial infection certain other medicines as recommended by a doctor are useful. Get a vaginal swab for culture sensitivity done. There is a great need of cleanliness of the genital area during pregnancy.

The following are some of the common warning signs during pregnancy:

Warning Signs	Possible Problems
Vaginal bleeding	• Miscarriage
	• Placenta previa
	• Premature labour
Abdominal pain	• Ectopic pregnancy
	• Premature labour contractions
Leakage of fluid from the vagina	• Rupture of membranes
Puffiness or swelling of face, hands and feet	• Preeclampsia (toxemia)
Severe persistent headache	• Preeclampsia (toxemia)
Pain/ burning sensation while urinating	• Urinary tract infection
	• Sexually transmitted disease
Irritating vaginal discharge, genital sores or itching	• Urinary tract infection
	• Sexually transmitted disease
Nausea	• Hyperemesis gravidarum
	• Infection

Leucorrhoea (vaginal discharge)

The secretions from the uterus and the upper portion of the vagina flowing down are reabsorbed in the lower part of the vagina. This is the normal, constant flow within the female organs. The presence of infection in any of these tissues usually causes a whitish discharge (called leucorrhoea). This white or pale watery discharge accompanied by pus may arise from *trichomonas vaginalis*, an infection due to a small parasite that normally inhabits the bowel. Other reasons could be pelvic congestion, endocrine disturbances, lacerations, injuries, perhaps atrophy of the vaginal tissues (following the menopause), an irritation of the labia or soiled undergarments, dirt, intestinal worms and masturbation. Excess secretion is expected when the girl reaches puberty due to over activity in her sex glands and organs. Some young women have a slight discharge at the time of ovulation, but this is not abnormal, nor does it indicate the presence of any disease.

In mature women, a profuse yellowish discharge accompanied with burning sensation and intense itching while urinating may be due to a serious infection–gonorrhoea. A thin, watery discharge may be due to the presence of cancer in the uterus or cervix, whereas a creamy discharge, slightly blood-stained may be due to trichomonas or some infection. From the early pregnancy period to mid forties, infections may sometimes follow the birth of a child because of the cervix being damaged during the delivery of the baby. Unless properly treated, infection may continue to spread to the other areas of the genital tract, even leading to cancer. A Pap smear, blood test and the skin test should always be done if there is a yellowish discharge. The following measures are taken to treat leucorrhoea:

- Doctors usually suggest strong antibiotic treatment to subside the infection.
- Take a vinegar douche. Mix two tablespoons of vinegar to a quart of warm water. After douche, a vaginal suppository or tablet should be inserted in the vagina.
- For severe itching, triple sulphonamide cream may be applied inside the vagina to control the infection.
- Cream containing the hormone estrogen, applied locally will benefit.
- For a more persistent infection of the cervix, electric cauterisation may be necessary, followed by a vinegar douche each night.
- In any persistent case of female infection, the husband should be carefully examined and treated for any infection. The treatment should be taken strictly under the supervision of a doctor.
- A leucorrhoea patient should undertake regular exercises like running, playing and do household work.
- Take every morning a dose of dried and powdered bark of the *mulsari* tree (*minusops elengi*) mixed to an equal quantity of brown sugar and water in consultation with a naturopath.

- Don't stay up till late at night and also avoid sexual intercourse during the course of the disease.
- Avoid fried, spicy foods and pickles.

Recommended yogic exercises are – *bhunamanasana, shalabhasana, ek pada uttanasana, vakrasana, suptavirasana* and *mulabandhasana.*

Bhunamanasana

Bhunamanasana allows the leg muscles to be elongated, spinal column to be stretched and sympathetic nerves to be massaged. Sit in dandasana and spread the legs on both the sides as much as you can. Hold the toes and lower the upper body. Touch the nose to the ground. The buttocks should not rise off the floor. Straighten the trunk and return to the forward facing position.

This asana stretches the leg muscles and the spinal column.

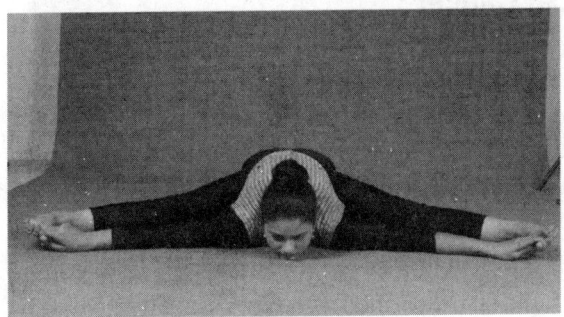

Bhunamanasana

DISEASES OF THE CERVIX

Intra-epithelia Lesion

It consists of carcinoma in the cervical generally in the reproductive age. The disease is associated with conditions like vaginitis, cervicitis and cervical dysplasia. Important measures to treat the disease are:

- Pap smears examination at an interval of 4 to 6 months.
- Cryotherapy.
- Electrocautery and electro-surgical loop excision.
- Laser ablation or conisation.

Carcinoma in the Cervix

The thickness of the epithelium is replaced with invasive carcinoma usually occurring in early 30s. The prominent causes of this disorder are:

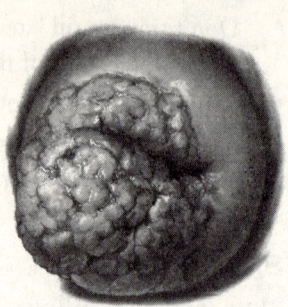

- Herpes virus
- Sexual activities at an early age
- Multiple sexual partners
- Use of oral contraceptives

Carcinoma in the Cervix

- Early childbearing

Important measures to treat the disease are –

- Standard hysterectomy, ablation therapy, cryosurgery and CO_2 laser therapy.

Cervical Cancer

Almost all cancers of the cervix are carcinoma. Cervical cancer is common in women between 40 to 60 years of age. It is generally caused by the following reasons:

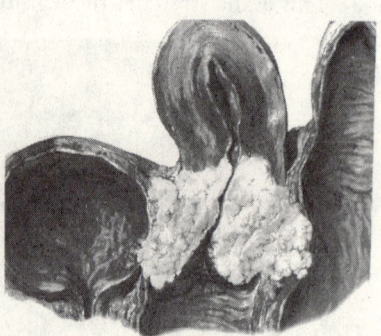

- Early sexual activities
- Multiple sexual partners
- Presence of sexually transmitted viral infections.

Signs and symptoms of the disease include: *Cervical Cancer*

- Abnormal Pap smear
- Dark vaginal discharge
- Loss of appetite
- Bleeding lesion
- Swelling of legs
- Cervical polyp
- Vaginal bleeding
- Post-coital bleeding
- Weight loss
- Inguinal lymph nodes
- Cervical erosion

Chemotherapy is a curative measure to treat the disease.

Cervical Erosion

Cervical erosion is a normal condition that occurs when the squamous epithelial cells grow out of the cervix and form an inflamed, red velvet type area that looks eroded and infected. The causes of cervical erosion are –

- Severe vaginal infections or STD's such as herpes or early syphilis.
- Tampons.
- Insertion of a speculum or other objects into the vagina.
  The signs and symptoms of the disease are the following:
- Irregularly shaped lesions.
- Bleeding tissues resulting in post-coital spotting and increased discharge.
- Herpes simplex.
- Carcinoma under the epithelium surface.
- Suffering from syphilis (venereal disease), cervical polyp and cervicitis.

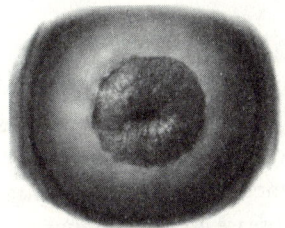
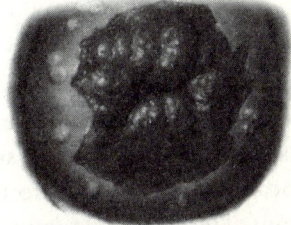

Congenital Erosion in Nulliparous Cervix

Effect of Hormonal Imbalance on Pregnant Women

Cervical Polyps

Cervical polyps are the fleshy tumours arising from the cells of the cervix generally in the age group of 40 to 50 in women having the history of the cervical infection resulting in inflammation. The signs and the symptoms of the disease include:

- Inter-menstrual spotting.
- Post-coital spotting.

- Smooth, soft, reddish purple to cherry red friable mass up to 4 cm in size at the cervix, which bleeds on slight touch.
- If neglected, there is a risk of cervical cancer, cervical eversion and cervical erosion.
- If not treated in time, this may result in conditions such as intra-menstrual bleeding, post-coital bleeding and leucorrhoea (white vaginal discharge). A Pap smear test is essential to examine the disease.

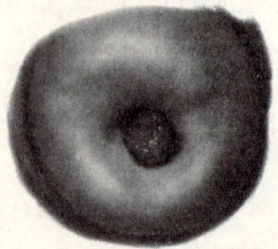

Small cervical polyp

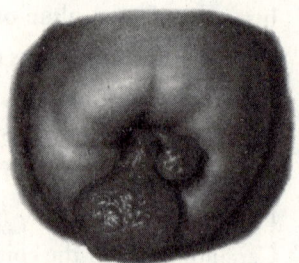

Large and small cervical polyps

Cervical Stenosis

Narrowing of the cervical canal may result in complete or partial obstruction during sexual intercourse and childbirth. The damage is caused by several reasons, such as cone-biopsy, electrocautery, cryocautery, radiation, infection and sometime due to congenital reasons. The signs and symptoms of this disease are the following:

- Pre-menopausal dysmenorrhoea (a sense of weakness and pain precedes the menstrual flow generally due to irritation in the ovaries).
- Abdominal bleeding
- Infertility
- Uterine enlargement
- Post-menopausal asymptomatic

Dilation of the cervix under ultrasound guidance cures the disease.

Cervicitis

Acute or chronic inflammation of the endocervical glands or ectocervix usually during reproductive age and in adolescence usually caused by exposure to sexually transmissible infections, multiple sexual partners and herpes simplex disease. Signs and symptoms of this disorder are the following:

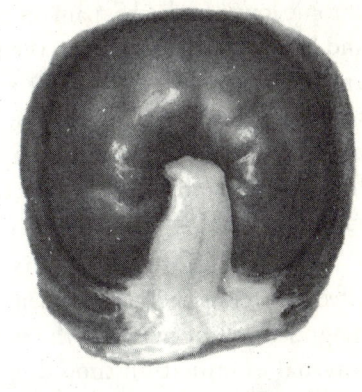

Appearance of cervix in acute infection

- Yellow discharge with white blood cells.
- Cervical erosion
- Post-coital bleeding
- Premature rupture of the membrane in pregnancy.
- Pelvic inflammation
- Premature labour and pre-maturity.

Seek the help of your doctor for treatment when the disease is diagnosed.

Nabothian Cysts

Retention cysts occur at the closure of a gland opening generally during the reproductive age. These are raised white, blue or yellow bumps ranging from 3 mm to 3 cm in diameter, which cause chronic inflammation of the cervix, followed by mucous-filled cysts and cervical cancer.

Infection of the Cervix

Infection of the cervix causes a condition known as cervicitis. Thrush and trichomonas are common vaginal infections, which attack the cervix and cause urethritis and cystitis. A thick yellowish and sometimes smelly discharge, which stains the underwear is the main symptom of a cervix infection. This is sometime accompanied with chronic lower backache, pain on deep penetration during intercourse and heavy bleeding between the periods. This disorder is common among women even in their sexually active life. It becomes a recurring condition sometimes. If the cervix is infected, then the fertility is often temporarily impaired because the sperms have to fight their way through the infection and the discharge on their way to the egg cell.

The infections of the cervix are not treated promptly and effectively either because women ignore the symptoms or the proper diagnosis is not made or the wrong treatment is prescribed. An internal examination should be carried out taking a swab and a couple of drops of mucus from the cervical canal. The treatment of cervical infection is given by pessaries, creams and antibiotics. The male partner should not forget to use condom when having sexual intercourse during the course of the treatment. Repeat the diagnostic tests after the treatment for few days to make sure that the infection is cleared up. The cervix, muscular in structure is the lower end of the uterus, which projects down into the upper part of the vagina. It has an opening or a canal leading to the inside cavity of the uterus, the glands of which secrete mucus. The cervix is capable of tremendous dilation and stretching when a closed canal becomes wide enough for a baby's head to pass through it at the time of delivery.

The cervix softens in early stages of pregnancy and hardens in menopause. Cervix, usually called the neck of the uterus is less than three centimetres in length and two to three centimetres wide. It is vitally important for good health, conception for maintaining a pregnancy and contributes to the normal delivery of the baby.

6

Yoga Asanas for Women

Ardha Chandrasana (the half moon posture)

Stand straight, arms sideways. Raise arms upwards. Bend right and raise left leg little off the floor. Return to the initial position. Repeat the posture on the right leg.

Benefits

- This posture softens the spinal column, lower back muscles and pelvic region.
- Slims down the hips, waist and thighs.

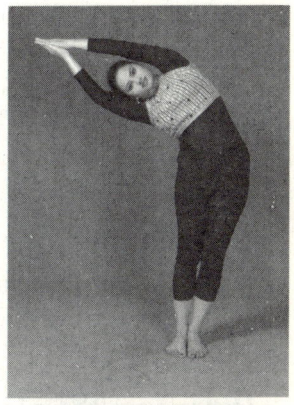

Ardha Chandrasana

Chakrasana (the wheel posture)

The body is made to look like a wheel in this yogic posture. Lie on your back and bring the palms under the shoulders. Raise the back and buttocks off the floor and curve the spine resting the crown of the head on the floor. Straighten the arms and arch and spine upwards as high as possible, lifting the head from the floor. Stay in this position for 6-8 seconds and return to the initial position slowly. Do not repeat this posture for more than two times.

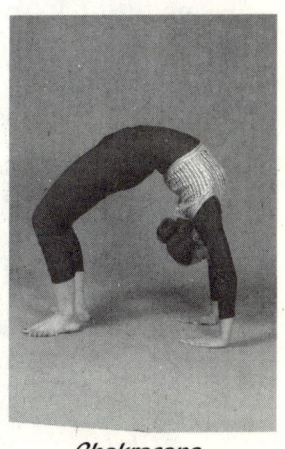

Chakrasana

Benefits

- Strengthens the muscles of the abdomen, thighs, shoulders and arms.
- Renders the spinal column flexible.
- Regenerates the kidneys.

Garudasana (the eagle pose)

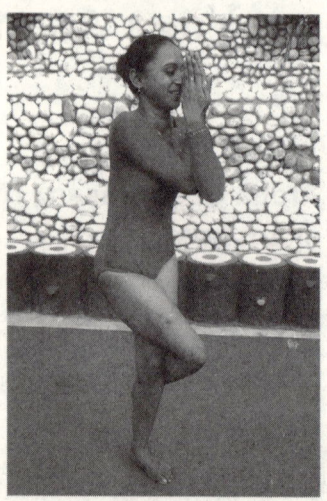

Stand straight looking ahead. Raise the right leg and twist it around the left leg. Now fold the arms and twist the right arm around the left arm until the palms are placed together to resemble an eagle's beak. Repeat this on the other leg as long as possible without strain.

Benefits

- This asana strengthens the muscles of the whole body and relieves cramps.

Garudasana

Halasana (the plough posture)

Lie on the back, arms stretched on sides. Slowly raise the legs exhaling and lower them behind the head until the feet touch the ground. Return to the starting position. Relax and repeat the posture. Avoid the strain in case of stiff spinal column.

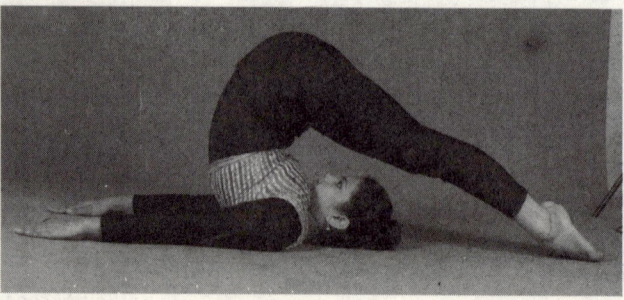

Halasana

Benefits

- This posture strengthens the glandular system.
- Keeps the genital and reproductive organs healthy.
- Relieves digestive problems.
- Strengthens the spinal column and back muscles.
- Relieves fat from the stomach, waist and hips.
- Helps curing tumours and sores in the vagina.
- Beneficial for persons suffering from low blood pressure (hypotension).
- Revitalises the nerves and muscles of the back.
- Removes exhaustion and fatigue.

Hasta Parshavasana

Lie on your back. Raise your arms and rotate them clockwise in circles behind the head. Repeat this exercise initially for 4-5 times and gradually increase it to 10 times.

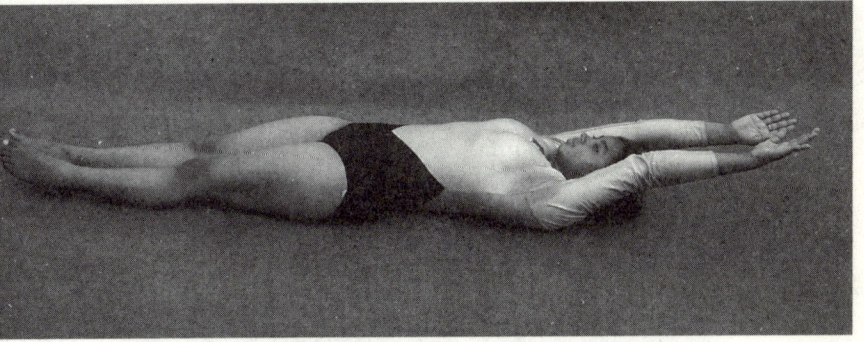

Hasta Parshavasana

Benefits

- This posture strengthens the muscles of the arms and the shoulders.
- It helps to enhance the beauty of the breasts especially if undeveloped or underdeveloped.

Janusir Merudandasana

In this posture, lie on your back. Lift the leg upward to enable the knee to touch the forehead. Stay in this position for 6-8 seconds and return to the initial position. Rest for 6-8 seconds and repeat this with the other leg.

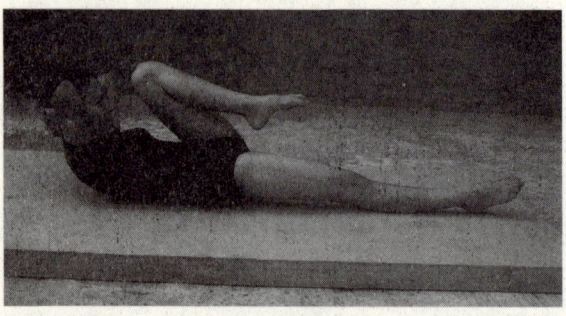

Janusir Merudandasana

Benefits

• The therapeutic advantages of this yogic asana are similar to *Janusirasana*.

Janusirasana (the head touching the knee position)

Sit on the floor. Bend the left leg touching the thigh of the right leg stretched in front. Bend forward till the nose touches the knee of the straightened right leg. Catch hold of the toe of the right leg with both hands. Stay in this position for 6-8 seconds, return to the initial position and repeat on the other leg.

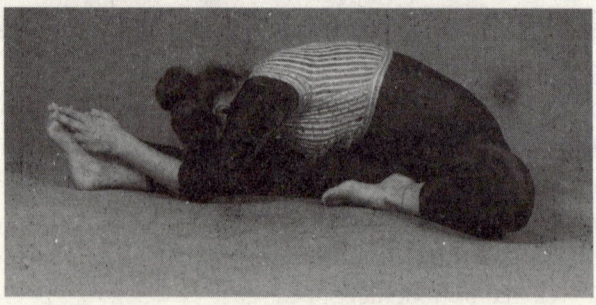

Janusirasana

Benefits

- This posture leaves beneficial effect on the nervous system.
- Makes the legs and muscles of the spinal column supple.
- Eradicates lines and wrinkles on the waist and the lower abdomen after the childbirth.
- Relieves dark spots and pigmented lines on the skin.

Kukkutasana

Sit in Padmasana with palms resting on the floor. Raise the thighs and hips off the floor balancing the body.

Benefits

- Strengthens the abdominal muscles.
- Helps to maintain the balance of the body.
- Strengthens the fingers, wrists, arms and the abdomen muscles.

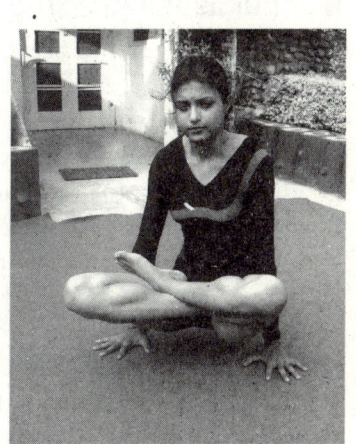

Kukkutasana

Malasana (the garland posture)

Sit on the feet. Lean forward placing the elbows and palms on the floor. Stay in this position as long as comfortably.

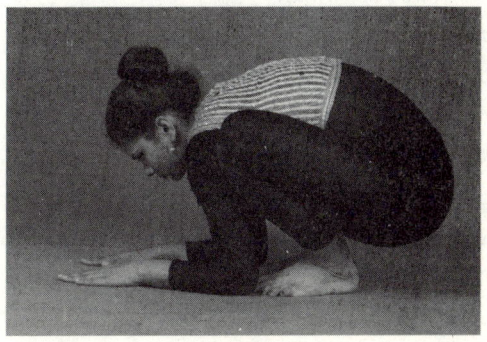

Malasana

Benefits

- This posture tones up the abdominal organs.
- Cures backache and all menstrual disorders.
- Makes the ankles flexible.
- Controls the malfunctioning of ovaries which causes excessive bleeding during periods.

Mandukasana (the frog posture)

Sit on folded legs and breathe normally. Do not proceed in case of pain. Supporting the body weight separate the knees, gradually moving the left knee further to the left side and right knee to the right side separating them as much as possible comfortably. Put the hands on the thighs. Breathe normally and stay in this position for 8-10 seconds and return to the original sitting position. Repeat this asana 4-5 times.

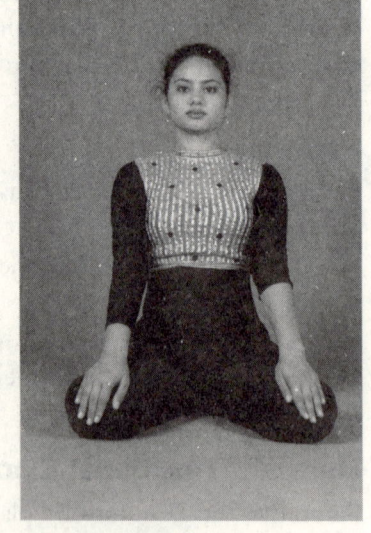

Mandukasana

Benefits

- Slims the thighs and hips.
- Enhances sexual potential.
- Cures cramps and varicose veins in legs.
- Helps curing displacement of the uterus.
- Corrects all the disorders of the reproductive organs.
- Strengthens muscles and nerves of the lower part of the body.
- Cures piles and improves the digestive system of the body.
- Increases blood circulation to the stomach and reduces fat from the thighs, hips and abdominal areas.

Matsyasana (the fish posture)

Sit in padmasana. Inhale, then exhale and lean the trunk backwards. Lift the chest upwards resting the crown of the head on the floor. Hold the position for 60 seconds, return to the initial position and repeat the posture 3-4 times. When performing this posture press the thighs and knees to the floor keeping the legs crossed.

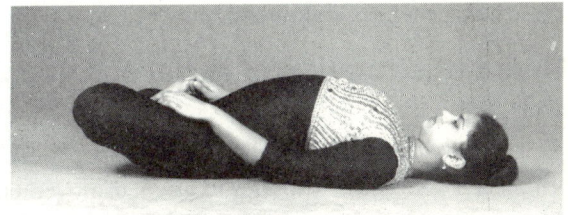

Matsyasana

Benefits

- Strengthens and regenerates thyroid glands.
- Strengthens the spinal column.
- Promotes the flow of blood to the entire body.
- Keep the abdominal organs healthy.
- Fortifies the muscles of the back.
- Refreshes the body and the mind.

Natrajasana

Stand up on the right leg and fold back the left leg at the knee. Grab the toes of the left leg with the left hand. Raise the right hand in front and try to see the top of right hand. Stay in this position for 8-10 seconds and breathe normally. Return to the standing position and repeat this on the other leg. Avoid doing this asana for more than six times a day.

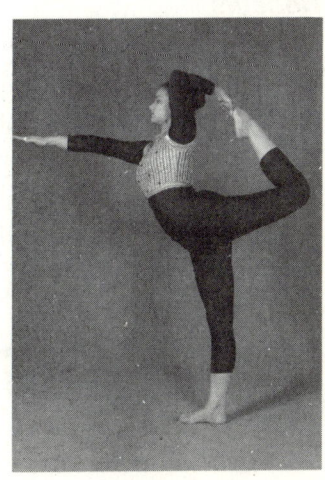

Natrajasana

Benefits

- This posture regenerates vigour, vitality, potency and beauty.
- Removes spinal disorders, enhances the digestive power and improves the eyesight.
- Strengthens the bones in the body.
- Makes the spinal column strong and supple.
- Strengthens/regenerates abdominal muscles.

Nauli Mudra (the rotation of rectal and abdominal muscles)

This posture can be practised in standing or sitting position by slowly rotating the rectal abdominal muscles in circular movement. Lean forward slowly towards the right and press hard on the right thigh with the right hand leaving the left hand loose.

Benefits

- This yogic posture strengthens and regenerates abdominal muscles and organs.

Ourdhva Paschimottanasana

The procedure of this yogic posture is similar to paschimottanasana.

Benefits

The therapeutic advantages of this asana are also similar to paschimottanasana.

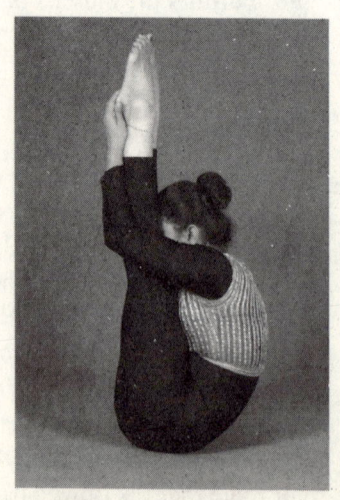

- Extremely beneficial for the facial skin, scalp disorders and hair.
- Helps relieve disorders of genito-urinary and reproductive organs.
- Cures constipation.
- Strengthens abdominal muscles
- Benefits the spinal column. Prevents the formation of fat around the stomach.

Ourdhva Paschimottanasana

Parivritta Janusirasana
(the spiralled head to knee pose)

Sit on the floor keeping the right leg flat on the floor. Lean your body to the right side and touch the right feet with both hands. Remain in this position for 10 seconds. Return to the initial sitting position and repeat the posture on the other side.

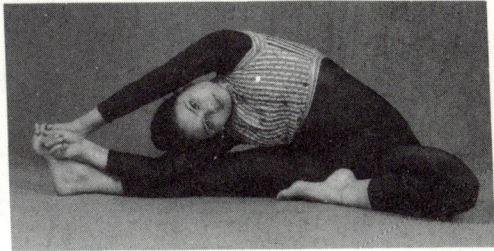

Parivritta Janusirasana

Benefits

- This yogic posture tones up the circulation around the spinal column.
- Soothes backache.
- Eradicates lines and wrinkles on the lower abdomen after childbirth.
- Eliminates excess fat around the abdomen, waist and hips.
- Benefits the nervous system.

Pasasana (the chord posture)

Sit on your feet as if on the toilet seat. Take both the arms on the back and catch hold of the fingers.

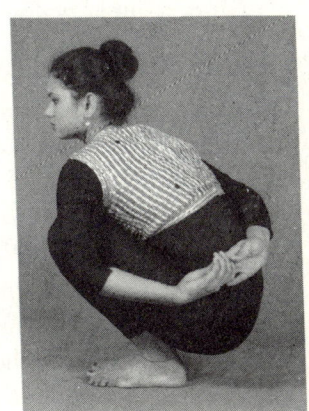

Benefits

- Benefits the spinal column, liver, spleen and pancreas.
- Helpful in menstrual irregularities.
- Relieves itching pain in the vagina.
- Rids extra fat around the waist, stomach and hips.

Pasasana

Paschimottanasana (stretching the back and legs)

Sit down with both the legs extended forward. Raise the arms above the head inhaling and lean forward until the head touches the knees exhaling. Hold the toes with your fingers. Stay in this position for 6-7 seconds and gradually sit up. Rest for 6-7 seconds and repeat 4-6 times.

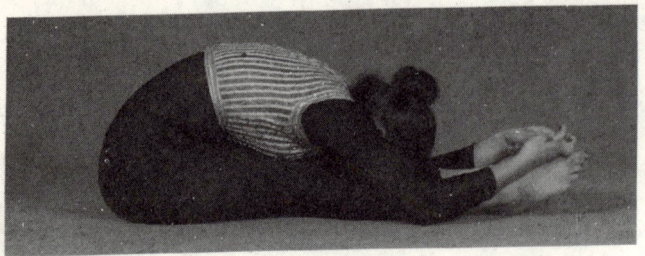

Paschimottanasana

Benefits

• Strengthens the organs of the abdomen, spinal column.
• Regenerates the kidneys and digestive organs.
• Relieves constipation and cures diabetes.
• Prevents the formation of fat around the stomach and back.
• Strengthens the reproductive organs.
• Stimulates the muscles around anus and pelvic region.
• Cures inflammation of prostate glands and uterus disorders.
• Cures respiratory disorders.

Pawanmuktasana (wind liberating pose)

This asana can be performed in standing as well as sitting position. Stand up with both arms hanging on the sides. Lift a knee up towards the chest without any pull on the ankles. Stand firmly on other leg. Stay in this position for 6-8 seconds and return to the initial standing position. Rest and repeat the posture on the other leg.

To do this asana in sitting position, lie on the back. The method of practice will remain same as in the case of the standing position. Bend your legs upto the chest and hold them tightly. Then lift your head up and touch your knees with the nose.

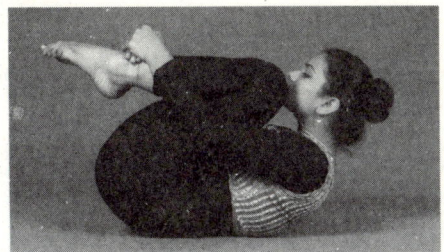

Pawanmuktasana

Benefits

- Strengthens the upper part of the body if performed during pregnancy.
- Helps the uterus come to its place if displaced during the delivery of the baby.
- Eradicates lines and wrinkles on the lower abdomen and waist after childbirth.
- Tones up the muscles of the abdomen and intestine.
- Cures constipation and gastric trouble.
- Corrects the malfunctioning of the stomach.
- Activates the pancreas and abdominal organs.
- Activates hormones producing glands.

Sarvangasana

Lie on your back and bend your knees towards the chest. Raise hips and legs off the ground supporting the back with your hands. Straighten the legs perpendicular to the floor. Stay in this position for 6-8 seconds and lower the legs slowly. Rest and repeat the posture 3-4 times.

Benefits

- Relieves headache, cold and cough.
- Cures constipation.
- Improves the functioning of all organs, glands and nerves.

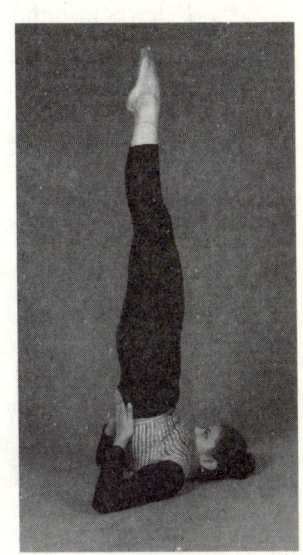

Sarvangasana

Setubandha Sarvangasana

This posture is a variation of sarvangasana in which the buttocks are raised from the floor and the back is arched.

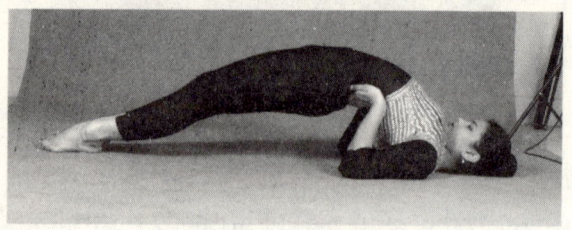

Setubandha Sarvangasana

Benefits

- Tones up the muscles of the back, spinal column, kidneys, legs and wrists.
- Refreshes the body and mind.
- Helps in the proper functioning of the thyroid glands.
- Regular practice relieves premature ageing. Helps to retain youthful vigour.
- Removes facial wrinkles.
- Relieves insomnia (sleeplessness) and depression.
- This posture is recommended to get rid of the habit of masturbation.

Shalabhasana (the locust posture)

Lie on the stomach with hands under the thighs and chin and forehead touching the ground. Stretch the legs and tense the arms.

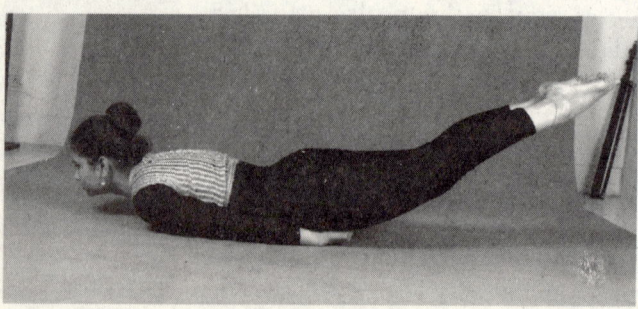

Shalabhasana

Raise the legs as high as possible comfortably. In case it is inconvenient to raise both legs, perform the asana raising one leg only. Hold the position for few seconds retaining the breath. Direct the attention to the upper region. Lower the legs, relax for sometime lying on the stomach. Repeat this asana for 3-4 times.

Benefits
* Strengthens the muscles of the back and abdomen.
* Leaves a beneficial effect on the digestive organs.
* Cures constipation and leucorrhoea.

Shavasana (the corpse pose)

Lie on your back and relax. Spread your legs apart. Close your eyes and let all the parts of the body relax. Breathe gently and observe your breath by concentrating on it. Breathe normally keeping the eyes closed and do not use pillow under the head. Shift your attention to the toes and concentrate on your feet.

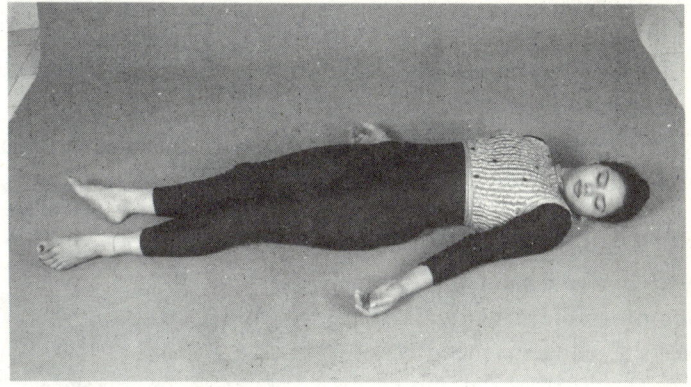

Shavasana

Benefits
* Relaxes all body muscles, nerves and organs.
* Helps those suffering from anaemia, hypertension, fatigue and heart disease.
* Relaxes the body.

Shirshasana

Interlock the fingers under the head. Slowly raise the knees and the hips off the ground and straighten your legs perpendicular to the floor. Initially take the support of the wall to do this asana.

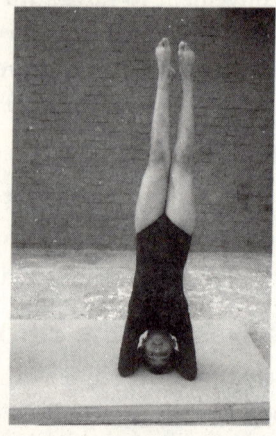

Shirshasana

Benefits

- Increases blood circulation in the upper portion of the body.
- Removes fatigue and builds up energy.
- Improves concentration and will power.
- Promotes growth and strengthens the entire body.
- Has a beneficial effect on the endocrine and digestive system.
- Increases facial beauty and cures facial skin diseases.
- Relieves fear, depression, mental tension, lack of self-confidence, disturbed sleep and nightmares.
- Improves the functioning of the sex glands and enhances sexual potentiality.

Simhasana (the lion pose)

Sit in padmasana. If you feel uncomfortable, sit in vajrasana. Place the palms on the knees and press the buttocks downwards. Open the mouth wide and stretch the tongue out downwards towards the chin. Gaze at the tip of the nose.

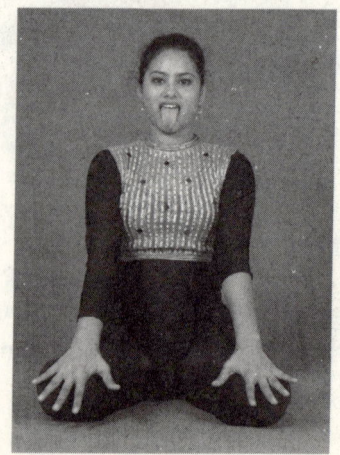

Benefits

- The practice of this asana is very beneficial for pregnant women.

Simhasana

- Helps get rid of bad breath, cures throat troubles.
- Has a good effect on the respiratory system and makes the lower spine elastic.

Supta Vajrasana (the supine pelvic posture)

Sit on the ground on your heels. Lean backwards slowly until the back and the head rest on the ground. Place hands under the nape of the neck. Relax the body completely for some time and then get up with the support of the elbow. Repeat the exercise 3-4 times.

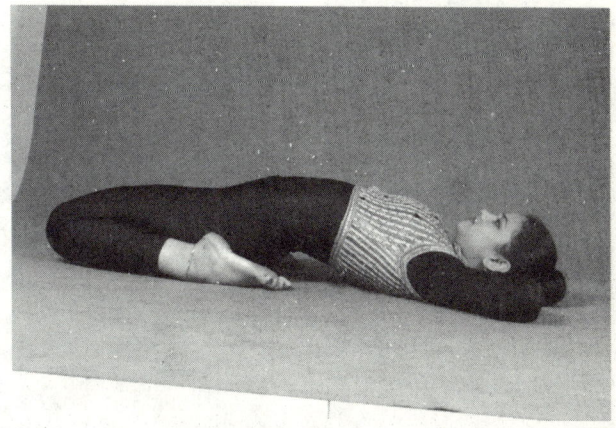

Supta Vajrasana

Benefits

- This asana increases the vital energy, increases the flow of the blood in the nerves of the lower part of the body and cures constipation.
- Stimulates muscles of the ankle, knees, legs, thighs and trunk.
- Helpful if suffering from epilepsy and piles.
- Cures indigestion and wind trouble.
- Energises the whole body.
- Increases the flow of blood in ankles, legs, thighs, hips, trunk and the lower part of the body.

Tarasana (the heavenly stretch pose)

This yogic posture has three positions. Stand straight. Raise both arms to the shoulder level and hold for 10-15 seconds. This is position No. 1. Now raise the arms straight over the head and hold for 10-15 seconds. This is position No. 2. Finally bring both hands on sides and hold for 10-15 seconds. This is position No. 3.

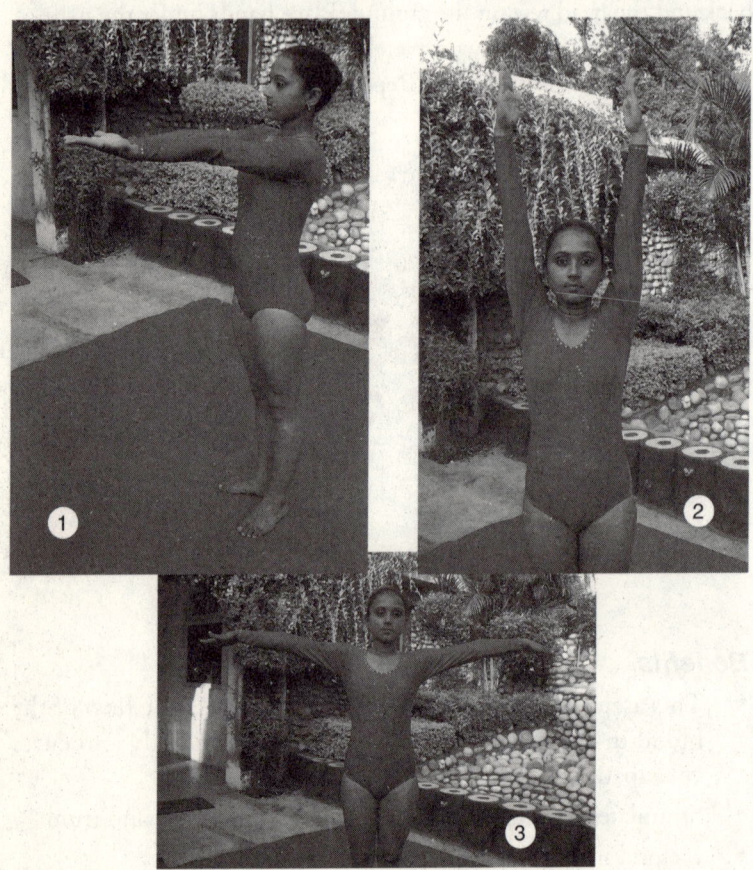

Benefits

• Beneficial for women during pregnancy and after the childbirth to keep themselves fit.

• Strengthens the lungs, chest and the respiratory system and cures asthma.

Trikonasana
(the triangle posture)

Stand with your legs apart. Raise hands to shoulder level at the sides. Slowly bend towards the left leg, touch the toe with the right hand, keeping the knees straight. Raise the left hand up and focus the gaze on the fingers of the left hand.

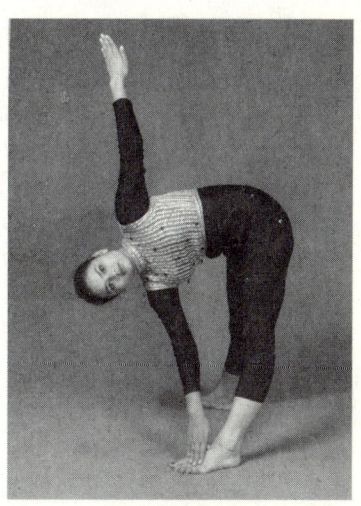

Trikonasana

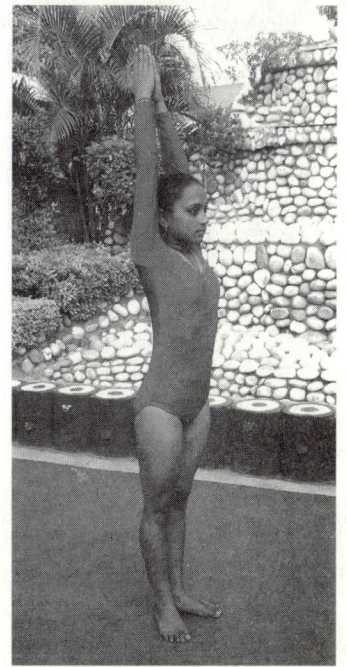

Urdhva Hastasana

Urdhva Hastasana

Stand straight with equal weight on both feet. Raise your arms and stretch the arms over the head. Avoid protruding the buttocks.

Benefits

- This posture strengthens the back muscles.
- Makes the mind alert.
- It is especially beneficial for both mother and the baby after childbirth.

Utkatasana

Stand straight and stretch the arms upwards joining the palms. Bend knees as if sitting on a chair. Stay in this position for 5-6 seconds and return to the standing position. Repeat the posture for 6-10 times.

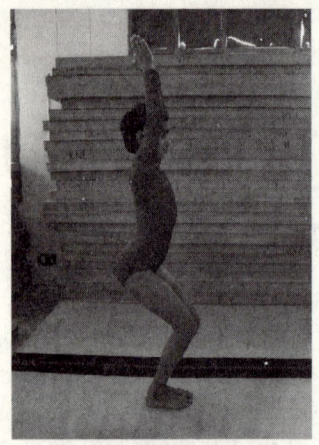

Benefits

*   This posture strengthens the nerves of the arms, legs, ankles, thighs and back.

Utkatasana

Viparitakarni Asana (the inverted posture)

Lie on your back and inhale. Raise the legs and hips with the help of your hands and exhale. The legs should form an angle of about 60 degree with the ground. Stay in this position for 6-8 seconds and lower the legs gently to the ground. Rest for 6-8 seconds and repeat this 3-4 times. High blood pressure patients should not practise this asana without consulting a doctor.

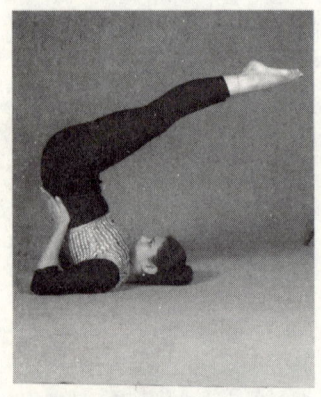

Viparitakarni Asana

Benefits

*   Revives the body.
*   Cures impotence (sexual weakness).
*   Relieves varicose veins, kidney complaints and high blood pressure (hypertension).
*   Relieves stress, strain and tension.
*   Revives the body.
*   Regenerates thyroid and pituitary glands.
*   Prevents the formation of facial wrinkles.

Vira bhadrasana (the warrior posture)

This yogic posture has three positions.

Position 1: Stand straight with arms on sides. Jump spreading the legs 3-4 feet apart. Raise both the arms up and bend the left leg to 90 degree and right to 45 degree. Revolve the hips and turn the trunk to the right. Return to the initial position and repeat the posture on the left side.

Position 2: Raise the right leg off the floor. Straighten the left leg and balance on it. Return to the original position and repeat the posture on the right leg also.

Position 3: Bend the left leg to form a right angle and look at the fingertips of the left hand.

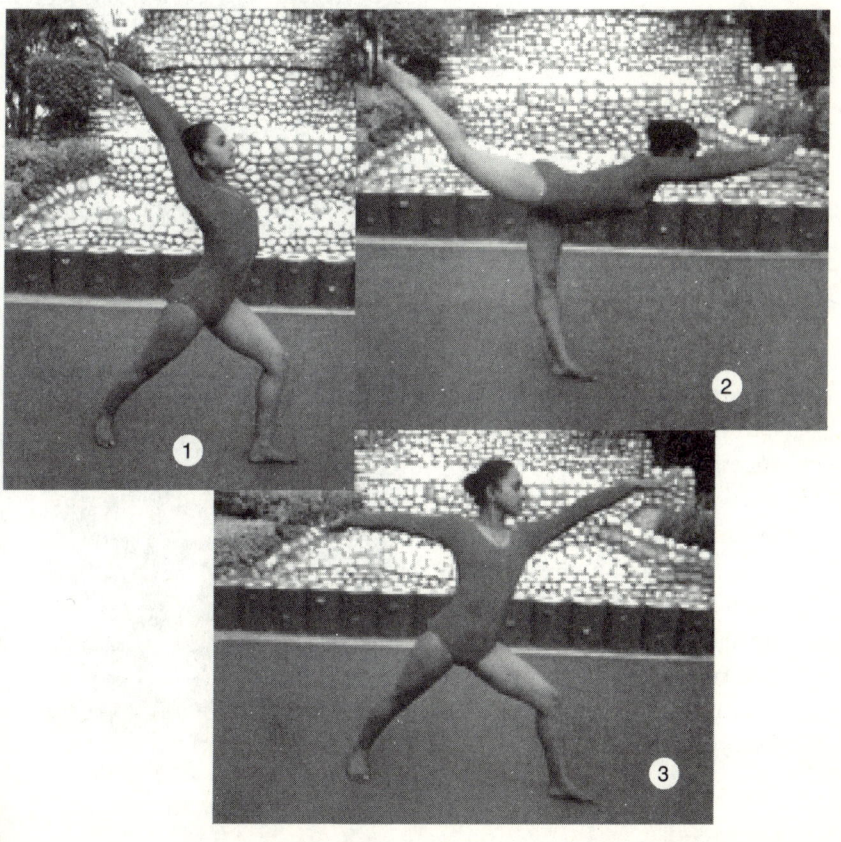

Benefits

- Builds up stamina.
- Improves balance and concentration.
- Strengthens the muscles of chest/ breasts, shoulders, back and stomach.

Vrikshasana

- Stand straight and stretch the arms up.
- Place the left foot on the right thigh and stay in this position for 10 seconds. Repeat the posture on the other side.

Benefits

- Improves concentration and balance.
- Strengthens arms, legs and shoulders and corrects the posture.

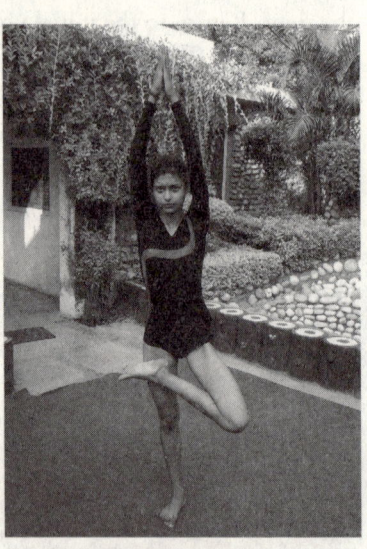

Yog Mudra (the symbol of yoga)

Sit in padmasana. Take your hands behind and hold them together. Lean forward slowly until the forehead touches the ground. Stay in this position as long as you can comfortably without breathing. Now sit upright and relax. Repeat this 3-4 times. Avoid straining or jerking the spinal column when leaning forward.

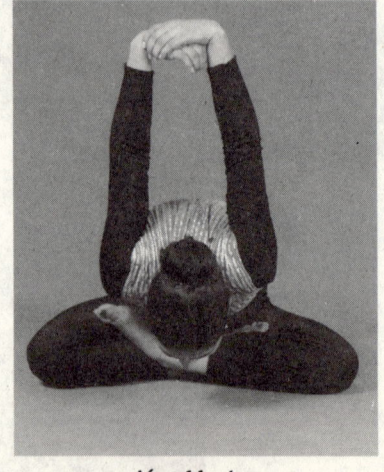

Yog Mudra

Benefits

- Cures white vaginal discharge.
- Benefits in case of premature separation of the placenta.
- Cures kidney complaints.
- Tones the abdominal muscles.
- Exercises the lungs.
- Helps the flow of blood from the lower region of the body to the upper.
- Has a curative effect in asthma.
- Corrects the disorders of the spine and strengthens the digestive system.
- Enhances sexual potentiality.

7

Natural Remedies for Some Common Women Diseases

Asthma

Asthma is a chronic and complicated disease women often suffer from. It has the following symptoms:

- Breathlessness
- Severe coughing and wheezing
- Tightness in the chest
- Excessive yawning or extreme fatigue

In nearly 80% cases below 40, asthma is triggered by:

- Allergy, such as grass pollens, animal hair or dust mites.
- An improper diet that lacks all required nutrients.

After the age of 40, in over 50% cases, asthma is caused due to lung infections or disorders such as emphysema. Asthma patients are advised by the doctor to use inhaler immediately when having an asthma attack. If still there is difficulty in breathing after using the inhaler, get in touch with the doctor. The following remedies help stop or reduce an asthma attack:

- Asthma patients should avoid smoking as far as possible. Sometimes, smoke in the house (especially in winter) worsens asthma. Asthmatics should not work on wood stove and chimneys while cooking.
- Asthma can be caused by stomach reflux in which acid backs up into the oesophagus from the stomach and drips down into the

breathing airway while sleeping. Prop the bed up and elevate the pillow while lying to prevent the dripping. Take an antacid medicine before sleep at night to cut down acidity.

- Stay indoors when it is too cold outside. Keep your mouth and nose covered with a scarf or mask while going outside.

- Breathe in a warm and dry climate.

- Magnesium is a useful mineral nutrient for asthma patients, which opens the bronchial tract–the airway to the lungs.

- Fatty acids reduce inflammation of the lungs during an asthma attack. Fish and flaxseed oil are rich sources of fatty acids.

- Swimming is an ideal exercise for asthmatics. Keep your mouth closed and breathe through the nose when swimming.

- Use auto air conditioning wisely as it brings the outside air which has pollens.

- Try to stay out of the kitchen as smelling the foods can bring an asthma attack.

- Beware of food additives that can trigger asthma.

- Use of the herb nettle relieves nasal allergies.

- Concentrate on breathing by drawing fresh air into your lungs, relax the body and control your anxiety – all these reduce the severity of asthma attack. Continue rhythmic breathing for 10 to 15 minutes.

- Have an anti-asthma diet. Fish, onions, ginger and garlic strengthen the immune system. Fruits and vegetables help control the free radical molecules in the body. Fruits and leafy green vegetables high in vitamin C and beta-carotene help fight inflammation. High fatty foods, and salt foods are unhealthy for people suffering from asthma. An asthmatic should eat more fish, drink milk and soyabean.

Pranayama

The yogic *pranayama* is an important respiratory exercise for asthmatics, which has been practised for centuries to control breathing. It is an act in which we inhale air from the atmosphere into our lungs, absorb the oxygen from it into our blood and exhale into the atmosphere along with carbon dioxide and waste water vapours. The process of inhalation and exhalation is repeated every 4 to 6 seconds and usually a person breathes about 15 times in a minute taking in nearly 500 ml of air.

There are three components of pranayama:

- *Puraka:* The act of inhalation in which the chest is expanded fully and uniformly without bulging the abdominal walls.
- *Rechka:* Slow, deep, uniform and controlled exhalation without bending the shoulders.
- *Kumbhaka:* Holding the breath in after puraka without straining the respiratory system.

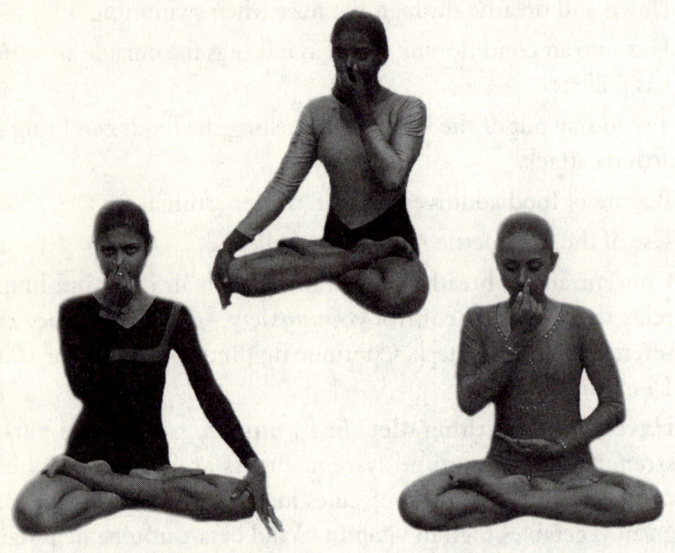

Pranayama

The Sanskrit word '*Prana*' means vital force or cosmic energy. '*Ayama*' means the control of the prana. Thus pranayama means the control of the vital force by concentration and regulated breathing – which is essential for life. The important postures for meditation or pranayama are padmasana, siddhasana, swastikasana, samasana, sukhasana and simhasana. Regular practice of these postures is beneficial for asthma patients.

Padmasana (the lotus pose)

Sit keeping the spinal column straight. Begin by placing the right foot on the left thigh and left foot on the right thigh resting hands on the knees. Fold your hands in *jnana mudra*. While practising take care not to hurt the genitals. Gradually increase the period of the exercise.

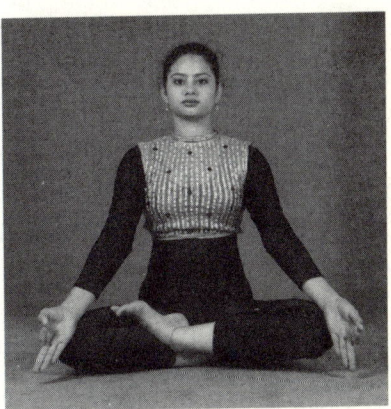

Padmasana

Benefits

*   This posture develops physical and mental stability and calms the nerves.

*   Relieves body stiffness and supplies blood to the entire body including the abdomen.

Siddhasana (the perfect pose)

Spread your legs forward. Place one heel at anus. Keep the other heel on the root of the generative organ. The feet or legs should be so nicely arranged that the ankle joints should touch each other. Hands can be placed as in *padmasana*.

Benefits

*   This sitting posture brings the body and spine into a balanced, erect and firm state and is ideal for meditation and pranayama.

Swastikasana (the auspicious pose)

It is sitting at ease with the body erect. Spread the legs forward. Fold the left leg and place the foot near the right thigh muscles. Similarly bend the left right leg and push it in the space between the left thigh and calf muscles. Now you will find the two feet between the thighs and calves of

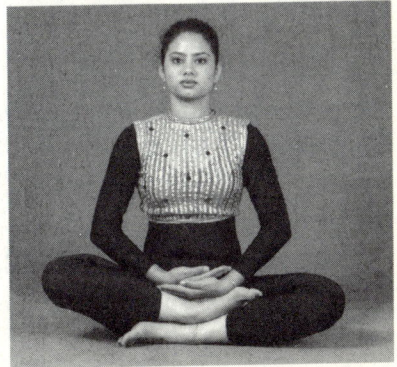

Swastikasana

the legs. Those who find it difficult can sit in *samasana*. The therapeutic advantages, however, are similar to the postures described above.

Benefits

- It improves one's concentrating power.
- This is a very suitable posture for knowledge, learning and meditation.
- It helps maintain normal temperature with in the body and tones the abdominal muscles and sciatic nerve.

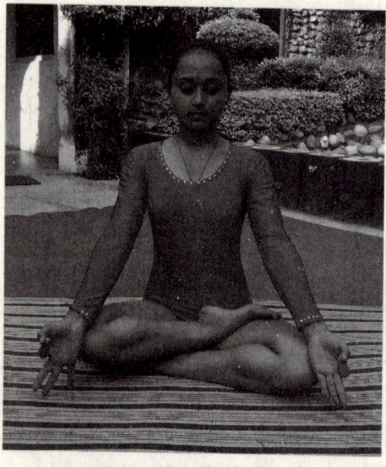

Sukhasana

Sukhasana (the comfortable pose)

Cross the legs, placing the feet below the knees. Rest the hands on the knees with palms facing up. Press the hip bones down into the floor. Breathe deeply through the nose down into the belly. Hold as long as comfortable.

Arthritis

Arthritis is a common ailment among women with the following primary symptoms:

- Pain
- Stiffness
- Swelling in and around the joints.
- Limited movement of the affected body organs.

There are several medical treatments (medication and surgery) to control arthritis pain but they are seen ineffective for permanent relief. Here are a few natural ways to cure arthritis:

- Control stress.
- Lose weight. The more overweight you are, the more stress and pressure you place on the joints of your body. This increases stress on the cartilage and bones.
- Eliminate food allergies that may cause this complicating disease.
- Remove toxic overload from the body.
- Learn to relax.
- Water exercises are excellent to relieve arthritis.
- Turmeric and ginger both boost the healing powers and reduce pain and inflammation of the arthritis.
- Use ice to prevent pain on the joints.
- Use heat to reduce the pain. When joints become hot, swollen and tender, heat is the best solution.
- Take fish oil capsules, which help in reducing the pain.
- Rub 'Mahanarayani oil' (readily available at any herbal store) on the area of pain, which brings immediate relief. But it is not a permanent cure. The oil penetrates the skin and softens pain-causing deposits in the bones.
- The herb *guggul* relieves arthritis pain, which travels to the arthritis bone and removes the imbalances causing stiffness, swelling and inflammation.
- Avoid vigorous exercises, which are unable to cure joint inflammation. Rather improve the time of the walk, physical activity and health status of the participant. Follow a light aerobic programme, cycling or swimming.
- Women usually put their baby on their joints, which is harmful in case of arthritis.
- Unfortunately, sleeping pills, tranquillisers and narcotic painkillers can become part of life for a woman suffering from arthritis, creating many problems than solving any. Consult a physiotherapist to recommend treatment to relieve the pain.
- Increase the intake of vitamin C. Lack of this vitamin can aggravate rheumatoid arthritis.

- Avoid hydrogenated oils, which interfere with the metabolism of fatty acids. These oils are found in margarine, peanut butter, most cooking oils and several other processed products such as potato chips, baked goods and salad dressings.
- In case of arthritis pain in hands and arms, which is common among women involved in household work, always massage the forearms from the wrists to elbows, using a compression technique.
- Vegetable juices (such as carrot juice, tomato juice, celery juice and cabbage juice) provide relief in arthritis. You may seek the advice of a doctor to suggest one suitable for you.
- Acupressure therapy cures arthritis pain and encourages the flow of the blood. It also helps to lubricate the joints, carry away toxins, reduces pain, swelling and inflammation.
- Yoga exercise is the key to restore health to the arthritic joints. The practice of yogic exercises such as *vakrasana, ardh badha paschimottanasana, ardh bhujangasana, supta vajrasana, bhunamanasana, pasasana, mandukasana, karnapidasana* and *parasarita pada uttanasana* are beneficial to relieve arthritis.

Ardh Badha Paschimottanasana

Sit in padmasana. Take the left hand behind the back and catch hold of the right big toe and with the right hand hold the left big toe. Look forward and bend forward resting the forehead on the ground. Return to the position of *padmasana* and repeat the exercise on the other hand. Repeat the posture 3 to 4 times. This posture is beneficial for arthritis patients.

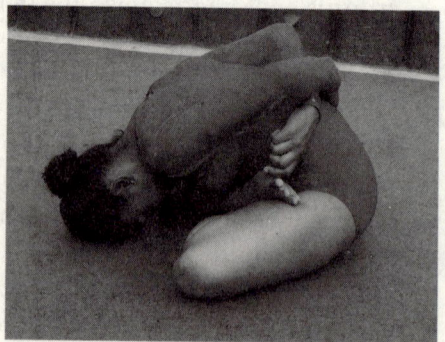

Ardh Badha Paschimottanasana

Benefits

- Cures premature separation of the placenta.
- Relieves all the problems faced by pregnant women.
- This asana if practised regularly can help in bringing the uterus and vagina in their original position after the delivery of the child.
- Makes the whole body supple.
- Develops the thoracic cage and improves the respiratory system.
- Effective against slow bowel movement.

Vakrasana (the spinal twist exercise)

This asana is similar to *ardha matsyendrasana.* Sit on the floor with both legs stretched in front parallel to each other. Keep the back straight. Let the right leg remain stretched on the floor and fold the left leg, taking it on the other side of the

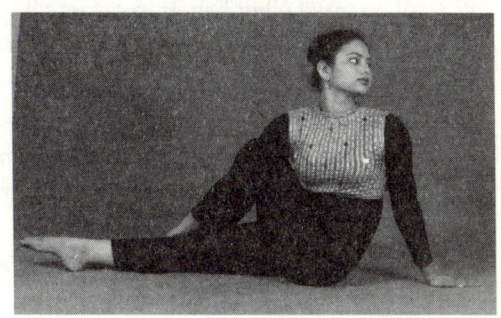

Vakrasana

stretched leg. Put the heel of the left leg close to the knee of the right leg. Start exhaling and turn towards left, keeping the neck and head stretched. Hold for 6-8 seconds and return to the initial position. Repeat this exercise on the other leg also. Do this 4-6 times alternately on each leg.

Benefits

- Relieves arthritis and stiffness in the knees.
- Leaves a curative effect on the spinal column, cures deformities of gall bladder, spleen, kidneys and bowels.
- Relieves constipation, stomach disorders, piles and backache.
- Has a good effect on the pancreas, adrenal gland, ovary in females and testicles in males.

Brown Spots

Brown spots are also called sun spots and are caused by the direct exposure to the sun's ultraviolet radiation damaging the colour producing cells of the skin. If the area around the spot has turned black and irregular in shape, then this is the sign of melanoma. Brown spots are a cosmetic problem, not a medical or health-threatening condition and can be removed by the following methods:

- Bleaching
- Liquid nitrogen
- Laser surgery
- Aromatherapy helps the spots to fade or lighten. Mix three drops of essential oil of lemon to carrier oil (preferably almond oil) and apply the mixture to the spot twice a day till the skin becomes clear.
- A mixture of honey and yogurt creates a natural bleach that can help lighten the spots. Mix 1 teaspoon each of plain yogurt and honey. Apply this mixture, let it dry and wash it off after half an hour.
- Yoga exercises such as *viparitakarniasana, sarvangasana, shirshasana* and *salamba shirshasana* enhance the circulation of the blood to the upper part of the body and are beneficial in case of brown spots.

Backache

Back pain, usually lower back pain is very common among women generally due to a ruptured disc or other spinal problems. Seek medical assistance in case of:

- Intense pain that travels down to legs or radiates from the spine.
- Sudden weakness in your legs.
- Loss of control over the bowels or bladder.
- Back pain that occurs suddenly without any reason.
- Back pain accompanied by fever, stomach cramps, chest pain and difficulty in breathing.

- Chronic pain that lasts more than two weeks without any relief.
- Acute pain that lasts for more than two to three days without any relief.

The following measures are taken to relieve back pain:

- Exercise is the best way to cure chronic back pain.
- Swimming is a great exercise for relieving back pain.
- Ice massage on the spot of pain for 5 to 10 minutes depending upon the condition helps to reduce swelling and the strain on the back muscles.
- Hot and cold treatment is the best way to relieve back pain. Do 15 minutes of ice massage followed by 15 minutes of heat treatment. Keep repeating the cycle.
- Stretching a sore back will enhance the healing process of backache.
- Sleep on a bed that doesn't sag in the middle when you sleep on it.
- Yogic exercises such as *bhujangasana, halasana, trikonasana, konasana, dhanurasana, chakrasana, malasana, trianga mukha ek pada paschimottanasana, shalabhasana* and *matsyasana* are beneficial in relieving backache.

Konasana (triangular posture)

Stand straight with feet 24 inches apart. Lean forward to touch the head to the knee of the right leg and hands held together behind on the back for 6-8 seconds. Return to the standing position. Rest for few seconds and repeat the exercise on the left leg. Perform this posture for 3-4 times on each side.

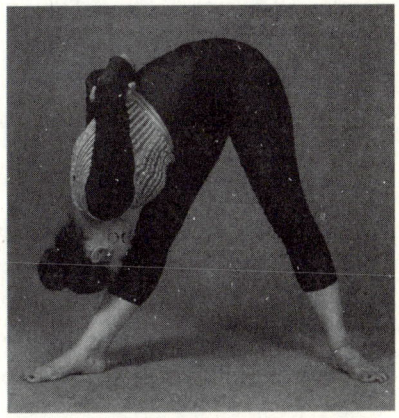

Konasana

Benefits

- Relieves backache and removes stiffness in the legs.
- Makes the spinal column and hip joints supple.
- Tones up the abdominal organs.

Trianga Mukha Ek Pada Uttanasana (intense stretch of the back)

Sit in Virasana. Bend forward touching the head to the knee of the stretched leg (right). Hold the feet with both hands. Do not tilt the body to any side.

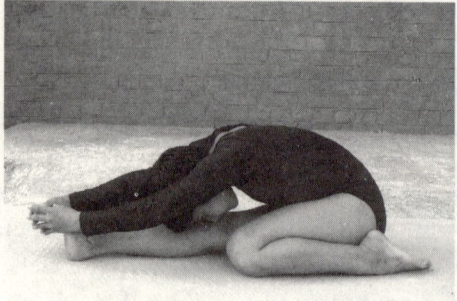

Benefits

- Relieves backache.
- Strengthens the muscles of the legs, hips, spine and abdominal organs.

Trianga Mukha Ek Pada Uttanasana

Knee Pain

Knee pain, a common disorder seen in nearly 40% women makes life miserable. Usually weight-bearing joints in the body make the knee – composed of two bones balancing on each other. Knee pain and swelling is a common symptom of this disorder. The following remedies are recommended to eliminate knee pain:

- Exercising on the floor eliminates misalignment that causes knee pain. Walking barefoot for five to ten minutes twice a day is an ideal remedy to cure the pain.
- Reflex therapy helps cure knee pain. Mix one drop of lemongrass essential oil with four to five drops of vegetable oil and massage gently on the affected area twice a day.
- All yogic exercises stimulating the nerves around the knee are beneficial to relieve knee pain or swelling.

Bladder Infection (urinary-tract infection)

Consult a doctor immediately if the following symptoms are observed:

- Blood contents in the urine.
- Fever and pain in one or both kidneys.
- Recurrent bladder infections in post-menopausal women due to hormonal imbalances.
- Frequent urge to urinate (cystitis).
- Burning, itching and painful urination.
- Nausea or vomiting.
- Pain in the lower back.

In nearly 30 to 40% cases, women suffer from bladder infections caused due to bacteria *E. coli*, which exists in the vagina. This bacteria makes its entry through the urethra (the tube through which urine flows). Between 15 to 20% women are seen suffering from recurrent infections. This disorder is more common among women with excessive sexual urge and the newly weds.

The following treatment is suggested for this:

- Keeping the vagina clean prevents the infection from recurring, which makes bacteria to move away from the vagina. Also keep the perineal region (between vagina and rectum) clean.
- Go to the bathroom before having intercourse, which helps to flush out the bacteria present in the vagina. Quite often the bacteria might be pushed into the bladder during an intercourse.
- Always go to the bathroom after the intercourse. Sometimes, bacteria at the opening of the male organ or at the opening of urethra gets way into the bladder. Urinary tract infections are more common in sexually active women and the sex act with such women leads to the accumulation of bacteria on the male organ.
- It has been observed that a bladder infection occurs in women involved in frequent sexual intercourse.
- Avoid douche as far as possible, which sometimes pushes bacteria into the vagina.
- Wear dry, cotton underwear. Avoid tight pants that reduce ventilation.

- Drink fruit juices and a lot of water to flush out the bladder and avoid infection.
- Vitamin C and vitamin A strengthen the inner surface of the bladder.
- Antibiotic drugs (recommended by the doctor) relieve infection. A daily dose of 1,000 to 4,000 milligrams of vitamin C and 50,000 international units of vitamin A is recommended, for which consultation with a doctor is must.
- Zinc strengthens the immune system and fights urinary tract infection.
- The herb, dandelion increases the flow of urine to help flush out bacteria, besides strengthening the immune system.
- If you develop honeymoon cystitis, usually a bladder infection occurs due to frequent intercourse. Consult a gynaecologist.
- Here is a natural way to get rid of the bladder infection. Lie on a slant bed and start rubbing your tummy just above the pubic bone for about 10 minutes. The massage improves bladder circulation and stimulates the flow of bacteria-ridden urine.
- Take hot bath in case of inflammation due to bladder infection.
- Women prone to frequent bladder infection should use pads instead of tampons during menstruation period.
- Yogic exercises such as *paschimuttanasana, vakrasana, ardha baddha padmasana* and *ardh matsyendrasana* are recommended in case of gall bladder disorders.

Ardha Baddha Padmasana (stretching the back and hips)

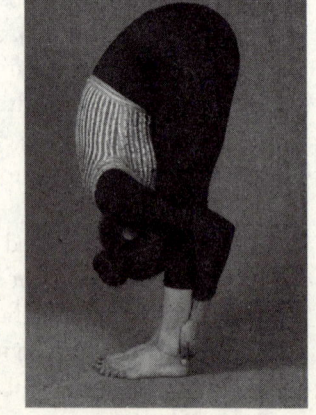

This posture can be performed both in standing as well as sitting position. Stand straight and raise both hands up. Bend forward until the head touches the knee. Take your hands at the back of your legs and hold them. Do not perform this asana more than three times. To practise this exercise in the sitting position, sit in padmasana. Raise the arms up inhaling, lean forward exhaling and touch the head to the knees.

Ardha Baddha Padmasana

Benefits

• Makes the back supple.

• Regenerates kidneys and abdominal organs.

• Relieves constipation.

• Stimulates the prostate glands, uterus and gall bladder.

• Prevents the formation of fat around the back, waist and stomach.

High Blood Pressure (Hypertension)

Between 50 to 70% women are seen suffering from a high or low blood pressure. If left untreated, blood pressure tends to rise slowly and steadily over a period of time.

Sometimes, a very high blood pressure strikes all of a sudden with diastolic pressure reaching over 130 mm Hg and systolic pressure to 250 mm Hg or even higher, which proves fatal. This condition is known as hypertension resulting in damage to the blood vessels, kidneys, eyes or brain. There are several powerful medicines for lowering the blood pressure. If the blood pressure is 160/100 or higher, there is need for pressure lowering drugs or natural remedies. To treat hypertension, following measures are helpful:

• Aerobic exercise for 30 minutes four times a week relaxes the muscles and decreases stress. It also helps to lose weight.

• Garlic eaten fresh or in supplement form helps lower high blood pressure.

• Avoid eating saturated foods, red meats and dairy foods. Non-vegetarians can have fish. Take seven capsules of high potency fish oil a day with the recommendation of the doctor.

• Fruits and vegetables high in potassium help to lower high blood pressure. Eat at least two bananas a day.

Low Blood Pressure (Hypotension)

For most of the women, the problem is not high blood pressure but rather low blood pressure, which may cause faintness when a woman stands for too long or indulges in excessive work.

A low blood pressure may cause:

- Weakness
- Fatigue
- Headache
- Fainting

In many cases, hypotension is caused by the medications a patient takes for hypertension, which include diuretics, alcohol, tranquillisers and antidepressants. The following measures are taken when suffering from a low blood pressure:

- Eat smaller, but more frequent meals.
- Sleep on a slant bed with the head of the bed elevated 8 to 12 inches above the feet.
- Talk less as far as possible.
- Avoid anxiety as one may faint.
- *Matsyendrasana* and *matsyasana* are important yogic exercises to control blood pressure.

Matsyendrasana

This yogic posture is similar to *ardha matsyendrasana* but is a little difficult to practise. The practitioner should begin with *ardha matsyendrasana* and gradually switch to *matsyendrasana*.

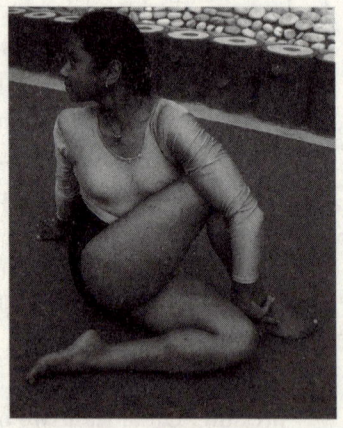

Matsyendrasana

Sit on the floor. Keep your legs straight. Fold the right leg at the knee and take it to the other side of the left leg. Start exhaling and turn the head, chest and waist towards the right side twisting the body as much as you can. Keep your back straight. Keep your right hand on the right side and with the left hand try to hold the right feet. Stay in this position for 6-8 seconds. Now start inhaling and return to the initial position. Repeat the exercise twisting the body towards the left side. Do this asana 4 to 6 times daily.

Benefits

- Has a good effect on the pancreas and glands such as adrenal, thyroid and sex.
- Corrects the disorders of kidneys, spleen, liver, stomach, intestine, bladder and pelvic and spinal region.
- Improves the blood circulation in the body.
- Beneficial for diabetic patients.

High Cholesterol

High cholesterol can be a serious health threat. Every woman should have her cholesterol level tested every six months. Cholesterol produced in the human body builds up new cells, produces hormones and insulates the nerves. A daily intake of cholesterol should not exceed 300 milligrams. High cholesterol level with mushy, yellow fatty substance circulating in the bloodstream is very harmful. It clogs the arteries and restricts the flow of the blood resulting in a heart attack.

The following measures are helpful to prevent the rise of cholesterol level in the body:

- Niacin, also known as nicotinic acid lowers the cholesterol in the body. The treatment should be taken up as prescribed by the doctor.
- Vitamin C and E raise the levels of protective HDL especially in elderly women. The cholesterol level drops by taking extra vitamin C. Citrus fruits, tomatoes, and strawberries are rich in vitamin C. Intake of vitamin E increases HDL levels and is very useful for people with high blood-fat levels.
- Calcium strengthens the bones and lowers the cholesterol level in the body. A study reveals 2 gm of calcium taken a day reduces cholesterol by 25% in a year.
- Watch your weight thoroughly. Your diet should consist of 2/3 fruits, vegetables, cereals and whole grains and 1/3 of calories should come from meat and dairy products.
- Cut fat from your diet, which can increase the cholesterol level in the body.

- Lemongrass oil, barley, rice bran help combat high cholesterol.
- Regular exercise and yogic postures decrease the buildup of cholesterol and help the body's ability to clear fat from the blood.
- Garlic and onions can reduce harmful blood fats.
- Cut down on beverages such as tea, coffee and avoid smoking cigarettes.

Dandruff (Seborrheic Dermatitis)

Scalp irritation, thick scales of dead skin, yellow crusting, red patches along the neckline and itchiness – these are the signs of dandruff. There are several causes of dandruff – a yeast infection of the scalp or hormonal imbalance. If the treatment to cure dandruff fails, consult a dermatologist for proper diagnosis and treatment. If you have dandruff do not apply anti-dandruff shampoo, instead treat your scalp with essential oils of aromatherapy. Dandruff is not a hair problem, but a skin problem. The flaking and itchiness are the result of the over-production of a substance called sebum, which is secreted from the sebaceous glands in the scalp. These glands are usually hyperactive because of excessively dry hair. Shampoos and strong medicines for the treatment of dandruff, however, may provide a temporary relief but they fail to treat the underlying disorders such as dryness and poor health of the scalp. Such anti-dandruff shampoos and strong medicines destroy the balance of water and oil of the scalp. The following natural remedies can stop flaking:

- Aromatherapy helps to eliminate dandruff. Mix 2 tablespoons of any mild shampoo, 10 drops of tea tree oil, 8 drops cedar wood oil, 6 drops each of pine oil and rosemary oil and 4 drops each of clary sage oil and lemon oil. These essential oils encourage the body's system to heal the problems causing dandruff. Tea tree oil is an antiseptic which helps to normalise the bacteria on the scalp. Rosemary and cedar wood oil increase circulation in the scalp. Pine oil encourages elimination of toxins from the scalp. Clary sage helps regulate and balance oil production and lemon eliminates toxins and promotes cleansing.

- Massaging the scalp twice a week with warm sesame oil combats excessive dryness. Massage the oil into your scalp before sleep for about ten minutes and wrap the head in a hot towel. Wash the hair next morning.
- Vitamin E helps to balance oils in the scalp and relieves dryness (recommended dose–a capsule of 400 international units a day).
- Zinc relieves dandruff. This helps to replenish the skin cells (recommended dose – 15-20 milligrams daily).
- Salenium relieves flaking and itching due to dandruff (recommended dose–200 micrograms supplement daily).
- Eucalyptus rinse helps fight infection due to dandruff. To make the rinse, put 4 teaspoons of dried leaves in ½ litre of boiling water, stir, remove it from heat, steep for an hour and strain the liquid. Add to it 1 tablespoon of apple-cider vinegar. After taking a shower, pour the rinse slowly over the hair and let it dry.

Depression

Depression is a common disorder among women. A depressed woman has the following symptoms:
- Sad or empty feelings most of the time.
- Feeling of hopelessness, guilt, worthlessness and helplessness.
- Loss of interest or pleasure in all activities including sex.
- Sleep disturbances.
- Loss of appetite and weight loss or gain.
- Decreased energy and fatigue.
- Restlessness and irritability.
- Difficulty in concentrating and making decisions.

Following measures are taken to treat depression:
- Get involved in physical activities and light exercises.
- Don't bottle up emotions within yourself.
- Avoid taking decisions during the period of depression.
- Yogic exercises like *setubandha sarvangasana* helps relieve depression.

Skin and Hair Problems

Oily Skin

An oily skin having medium to large pores on the skin has the following symptoms:

- Blackheads and acne
- Skin blemishes

To get rid of an oily skin following remedies are suggested:

- Aromatherapy treatments can be very beneficial for oily skin to help balance glandular activity, improve circulation and for detoxification.
- Steaming helps to deep-clean oily skin. Steam the face once a week. Start the face with cleaning, followed by steaming, rinse with warm water and finally splash cool water and pat dry.
- Yogic exercises such as *shirshasana, salambha sirshasana* and *viparitakarni asana* are recommended for healthy hair and beautiful skin.

Dry Skin

If the skin feels tight, looks dull and flaky, it is a dry skin. A dry skin is prone to wrinkles and premature ageing. If there is no improvement after two weeks of self-care, consult a dermatologist for diagnosis and treatment. The following steps should be adopted to treat a dry skin:

- Have a warm facial compress using essential oils. Lavender, rose or neroli are recommended essential oils to treat a dry skin.
- Do not apply soap to wash the facial skin. Use a washing gel.
- Apply moisturiser after the bath.
- Drink 7 to 8 glasses of water a day to keep the skin hydrated and to prevent dryness.
- Use oatmeal as a substitute for soap. Oatmeal is a soothing agent.
- Beta-carotene taken with lunch and dinner is a nutrient diet to keep the skin soft, smooth and healthy. (Recommended daily dose–15 milligrams a day).

- Zinc (recommended dose – 15 milligrams a day) is an important nutrient for the repair of damaged skin tissue. Zinc deficiency makes the skin dry.

- Vitamin B complex (recommended dose–100 milligrams a day) cures a dry or diseased skin.

- Vitamin C (recommended dose–1,000 milligrams a day) helps the immune system and leads to healthier skin.

- Vitamin E capsules (recommended dose–400 international units a day) help replace cells on the skin's outer layer.

Oily Hair

Hair become oily due to a high-fat diet. Sebaceous glands also produce oil known as sebum. A diet full of fried foods and saturated fats can trigger over-production of sebum. Women with fine hair have as many as 1,40,000 oil glands on their scalp. To get rid of oily hair the following remedies are suggested:

- Rinse the hair with lemon water after shampooing. Squeeze the juice of two lemons into two cups of soft water and apply it evenly on the hair and massage gently. Leave it on for five minutes and rinse with cool or tepid water. Blot the hair dry with a towel.

- Use of the herb horsetail is an effective remedy for oily hair. Boil one cup of distilled water and add to it 2 tablespoons of dried powder of horsetail. Use this as a last rinse after shampoo.

- Aromatherapy helps to cut oil in hair. Add 3 to 4 drops of rosemary, lavender, eucalyptus, cypress or lemon oil in water. All these oils are astringents and cleanse and tone the sebaceous glands.

- Massage your scalp while shampooing.

- Don't brush or comb your hair too much as it carries the oil from the roots to the ends of the hair.

- Learn to relax. When you are under stress, the body produces more androgens, which produce excessive oil.

- Apply astringent to the scalp, which helps slow down oil secretion from the scalp.

Dry Hair

Like skin, hair look lifeless if they lack lustre, are dry and brittle with split ends. Hair become dry as a result of too much exposure to the sun, blow drying or chemical treatments including colouring and perming. Use hair conditioner to lubricate the hair and to prevent static electricity. Beer can be used to give a crisp, healthy, shiny look to dry hair.

Salambha Shirshasana (head stand pose)

Salambha shirshasana is an advanced form of *shirshasana* which is also called "The King of Yoga Postures". Kneel in front resting the forearms on the ground and slowly raise the knees, hips and legs off the ground till the legs straighten perpendicular to the floor. If you find difficulty in doing this asana, take the support of the wall. This is *shirshasana*. Hold for a while and bring both the legs horizontally parallel to the ground. This is *salambha shirshasana*.

Benefits

- Extremely beneficial for the facial skin, healthy growth of hair and for strengthening the muscles of the entire body.
- Cures menstrual disorders.
- Enhances sexual prowess in women.
- Helps in curing the disorders of genito-urinary and reproductive organs.

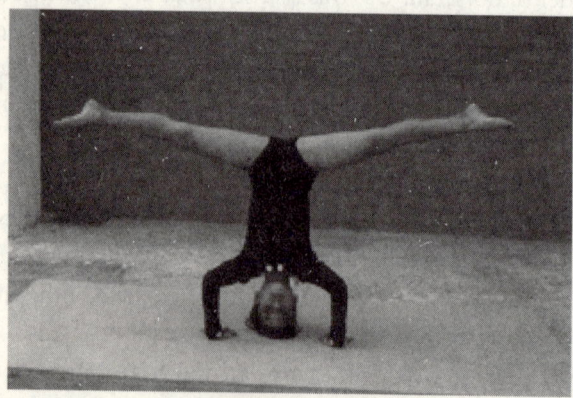

Salambha Shirshasana

Hair Loss

Hair loss in women is caused by many reasons as below:

- Alopecia areata (baldness on the scalp in patches).
- Hormonal imbalance.
- Menopause.
- Shortage of dietary protein or amino acid deficiency.
- Intestinal parasites.
- Hair treatments generally due to chemical hair dyes or perming lotion.
- Stress or sudden shock.
- After-effect of high fever.
- After childbirth.

Following measures are suggested to stop hair fall:

- Consult a doctor for suitable treatment, if hair continue to fall even after a treatment.
- Aromatherapy is an important measure to stop hair fall. Essential oils of jojoba, rosemary, lavender, lemon balm and cedar wood help fight hair loss. Massage these essential oils into the scalp with your fingertips. Leave it on for minimum 45 minutes or overnight and shampoo in the morning. Add one drop each of lavender oil and rosemary oil to ½ litre water and pour it over the head as a final rinse.
- *Viparitakarniasana, shirshasana, salambha shirshasana, parasarita pada-uttanasana* and *ushtrasana* are important yogic postures to help the growth of hair.

Fatigue

In today's busy and stressful life, fatigue among women is a common problem. The following conditions can cause very serious fatigue:

- Low thyroid function
- Mononucleosis
- Illness including hepatitis, thyroid diseases and cancer
- Overwork

The following measures prove helpful to fight fatigue:

- Eat foods and drinks that provide you high-octane energy fuel. Avoid high-fatty foods in the evening.
- Have sufficient rest. Try to go to bed early and get up at the same time every day.
- A good restful sleep in a cool, dark and quiet room relieves fatigue. Sleep on your side for easier breathing.
- Warm up exercises for 10 to 15 minutes in the morning before starting the day are very beneficial.
- Eat sufficient carbohydrates, proteins and fats in your breakfast to control and over-activate your insulin and blood sugar.
- Do not have coffee after a meal, as it can disturb sleep.
- A brisk walk for 10 minutes can energise you for hours. It also tones up your muscles.
- Gentle yogic exercises help build your energy.
- Avoid watching TV as far as possible, as it makes one lethargic. However, reading helps to energise.
- Think positive, be motivated and confident. These thoughts affect your energy level.
- Breathe deeply, that makes you relaxed and energised.
- Avoid taking sleeping pills as they are harmful.
- The colour on the walls of your house leaves a good effect on your mind. Dark colours make you feel fatigued. Red colour is good for short-term energy stimulation. Green colour is good for eliminating fatigue.
- Light music helps fighting fatigue.
- Yogic exercises such as *shirshasana, salambha shirshasana, parasarita pada uttanasana, karna pidasana* are helpful in relieving fatigue.

Parasarita Pada Uttanasana

'*Parasarita*' means spread, '*Pada*' means legs and '*Uttana*' means intense. Stand erect, spread the legs 3 to 4 feet apart, toes pointing forward. Bend down keeping the legs straight and place your palms on the floor. Rest the crown of your head on the floor. Hold for sometime and raise the head.

Benefits

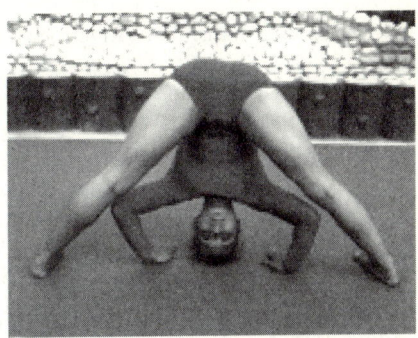

Parasarita Pada Uttanasana

- This asana relieves aches and cramps in the calves.
- Cures all menstrual and genital disorders in women
- Eradicates fatigue.

Karna Pidasana

Perform halasana. Now bend the knees resting them on the ground close to the ears. Hold your calves with both hands.

Benefits

- Helps relieve fatigue and cures all digestive problems.
- Keeps the spinal column supple and healthy.

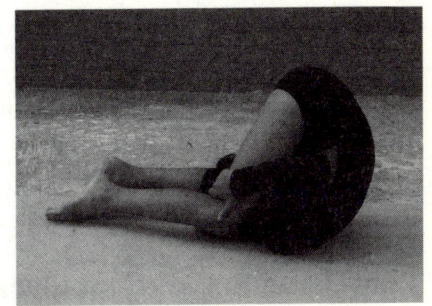

Karna Pidasana

- Revitalises the nerves and muscles of the back and removes exhaustion.
- Relieves obstruction of urine and prevents fat from forming on the stomach, hips and waist.

Gout

Gout is a type of arthritis that causes severe pain, often striking at night. The skin of the affected joint (mostly big toe) becomes red, sore, swollen and tender due to the effect of uric acid crystals, which settle in the joints. Doctors usually inject toxic drugs to stop the pain by dissolving the uric acid crystals.

The following natural curative measures are suggested to treat gout:

- Apply crushed ice pack on the painful joint for about ten minutes.
- Avoid taking high protein foods and whole grain cereals that contribute to higher levels of uric acid.
- Drink a lot of water to flush out excess uric acid from the body.
- Avoid taking alcoholic drinks as they increase the production of uric acid in the body, which gets deposited on the joints.
- Eating cherries prevents the production of uric acid.
- Vitamin B6 helps distribute water in the body to keep all the tissues hydrated. This helps prevent uric acid turning into crystals.
- Take a tablespoon of apple cider vinegar in the morning daily to prevent gout.
- Mix ½ cup charcoal powder in the water and soak the affected foot in it for 30 to 60 minutes.
- Yogic exercises such as *utthita trikonasana, garudasana* and *ardha badha paschimottanasana* are beneficial to cure gout.

Low Blood Sugar (Hypoglycaemia)

This disorder causes several symptoms in women such as the craving for sweets, irritability, fatigue, dizziness, frequent headaches, poor memory, heart palpitations, depression and frequent anxiety or nervousness. The following curative measures are recommended to treat low blood sugar:

- Take a diet containing maximum protein but lesser carbohydrates. This diet should include white sugar and flour that strengthen the spleen and pancreas.
- Take a diet containing too much fatty, fibre free foods, red meat and too many refined carbohydrates.
- Taking vitamins, minerals and milk supplements to help cure hypoglycaemia.

Hepatitis C

A life-threatening liver disorder caused by viral infection, damages the liver or leads to cancer in women. A patient suspected to have hepatitis C should see a doctor immediately at the first sign of the symptoms, which include:

- An attack of fever due to jaundice
- Pain in the lower right side of the abdomen
- Loss of appetite
- Dark yellow urine
- Nausea
- Chills and fever

Few natural remedies for this disease are given below:

- Lemon balm: Add 1 teaspoon of dried or fresh herb to a cup of boiling water. Steep for 10-15 minutes, strain and drink (two to three cups a day).
- Garlic is an effective herb to treat hepatitis C. It can be taken in the form of capsule, fresh cloves or cooked. (Recommended dose – two to three capsules a day – 3000 to 4000 micrograms when prescribed by your doctor).
- Fatigue, nausea and diarrhoea are common conditions of hepatitis C. All these can be cured with acupressure treatment (pressing pressure points on feet and the waist). Consult a naturopath for treatment.
- Diets such as red meats (harming the digestive process, liver, gall bladder and pancreas), dairy foods (putting strain on the liver), alcohol, tea, coffee and colas that contain caffeine should be avoided.
- Drink distilled water as tap water contains chlorine, fluorides and inorganic chemicals.
- Fruit juices are high in concentrated sugar, which harm the liver and the digestive process of the body.

Yog mudra, vakrasana, bhujangasana, paschimottanasana, supta vajrasana, bakasana, mayurasana, pasasana, natrajasana and *pawan-muktasana* are the beneficial exercises for liver and digestive disorders and helpful in curing hepatitis C.

Headache

Headaches usually caused by muscle contraction have many types with symptoms of different health problems. The majority of headaches in women are known as tension headaches. Migraine accompanied by nausea and vomiting is the most common form of headache that most often strikes women with severe pain in one side of the head. Tension headache in the forehead causes dull pain on both sides of the head. There are many headaches that trigger from foods, stressful conditions and an imbalance of hormones usually accompanied by symptoms such as general weakness, dizziness, numbness, blurred vision and memory loss. Tension is the prominent cause of headache.

Skipping or delaying meals can cause severe headache due to muscle tension and drop in blood sugar level. High salt diets can cause severe migraine. Excessive noise triggers tension resulting in headache. Several factors such as proper diet and nutritional supplements, and stress management are recommended to cure headache.

Following remedies are recommended for the treatment of chronic headache as below:

- Exercise is a useful measure to prevent headache.
- Aspirin is an anti-inflammatory drug to cure headache but its overuse harms.
- Acupressure treatment of rubbing between the thumb and forefinger helps relieve headache. Pregnant women should not practise acupressure treatment because it may sometimes cause premature contraction of the uterus.
- Hot shower and applying heat on the neck relieves headache.
- Breathing deeply relieves tension headache.
- Tying a tight cloth (headband) around the head decreases the flow of blood to the scalp and relieves headache.
- Do not chew gum. It tightens the muscles causing tension and headache.
- Alcoholic drinks are harmful and cause headache.

- Avoid taking chocolate if prone to frequent headaches.
- Rub peppermint oil on temples. Dilute one part peppermint essential oil in two parts almond oil or any other carrier oil. Other essential oils such as lavender oil or roman chamomile relieve tension and cure headache.
- Vitamin B 6 stabilises the brain's serotonin preventing headache.
- Ginger water cures headache. Put a teaspoon of ginger in four glasses of water and drink it throughout the day.
- Constipation causes headache. Try to relieve constipation and change your eating habits accordingly.
- Low blood sugar triggers headache. To keep the blood sugar level balanced, have at least three meals a day.
- Regular practise of meditation helps to relieve migraine.
- Eliminate foods from your diet that seem to cause headache. Foods such as packaged meat and fish, vinegar, pickled and fermented foods, cheese, products high in yeasts (including coffee, cake and bread), citrus fruits, chocolate, sour cream and yogurt, caffeine and alcoholic beverages may sometimes prove harmful.
- Vitamin E (recommended daily dose 400 international units) helps to stabilise estrogen level and prevents migraine generally during periods.
- Calcium supplements can help decrease the frequency of menstruation, resulting in frequent migraines.
- Nearly 40% women having migraine as a result of hormonal changes during periods suffer low blood levels of magnesium, which generally causes migraines. Start taking 200 milligrams magnesium supplement a day and gradually increase to 400 milligrams a day. (You may consult a doctor).
- High altitudes trigger headache. Vitamin C relieves headache. Take 3,000 to 5,000 milligrams of vitamin C a day on high altitudes strictly in consultation with a doctor.
- Recommended yogic exercises to relieve headaches are *ushtrasana* and *viparitakarniasana*.

Ushtrasana (the camel posture)

To practise this posture fold the legs at the knees keeping them six inches apart and resting hands on hips. Stand on knees and let the ankles and toes of both legs fall flat on the floor. Curve back and catch hold of the soles of your feet. Remain in this posture for 10 to 15 seconds and return to the initial position. Repeat this posture for 3 to 4 times.

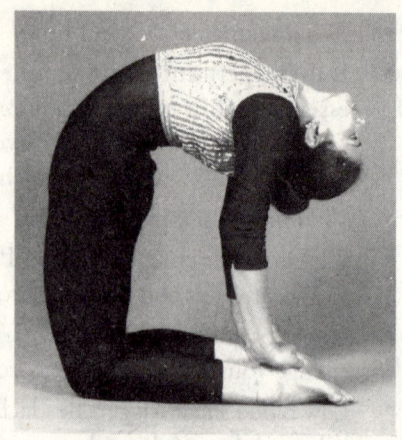

Ushtrasana

Benefits

• Cures chronic headache and visionary defects.
• Strengthens the muscles of the abdomen, spine, thighs, chest and arms.
• Removes stiffness in the neck and shoulders.
• Renders spinal column flexible and regenerates the kidneys.
• Corrects the whole respiratory system.

Leg Cramps

Leg cramps commonly occur in women often in late pregnancy while resting or sleeping. Cramps are usually caused by the following factors:

• Fatigue in the calf muscles
• Pressure on the nerves of the legs
• Impaired circulation
• Calcium-phosphorus imbalance in the blood

Cramps are relieved by the following measures:

• Stretch the muscles slowly and gently.
• Stretch the calf muscles gently keeping the knees straight, ankles bent and heels resting on the floor.

- A foot cramp usually tightens the muscles of the arch and curls the toes. Stretch out the toes to prevent cramp.
- *Gomukhasana* is a beneficial yogic posture to relieve leg cramps.

Cardiovascular Risk

Before having a heart attack usually the following symptoms are observed:

- Feeling of an uncomfortable pressure, fullness, squeezing pain in the chest generally lasting for few minutes.
- The chest pain spreads to shoulders, neck and arms.
- Feeling of light-headedness, nausea or sweating
- Shortness of breath
- Feeling of fatigue
- Difficulty in breathing
- Abdominal pain or indigestion

The following natural ways are beneficial to prevent the risk of a heart attack:

- A regular aerobics exercise programme 30 minutes a day strengthens the heart and lungs.
- Keep your cholesterol in control.
- Have a regular check over high blood pressure.
- Ensure regular check over your weight.
- In case of women above 50, vigorous exercises are not advised. However, they may involve themselves in moderate activities such as household work, morning or evening walk and gardening activities to improve fitness of the heart.
- Women who are physically unfit or above the age of 50 should check with the doctor before starting any exercise programme.
- Stretch for five minutes before and after the exercise.
- When feeling pain or pressure in the chest or along the left side of the neck, arm or shoulder, stop exercising and consult the doctor for thorough check-ups and tests.
- Light sports, jogging, cycling, skipping rope, walking, swimming and playing indoor games condition your heart.

- Heart patients should strictly avoid smoking. According to studies, every cigarette damages the lungs and shortens life by six minutes. A cigarette smoker has five times greater risk of a heart stroke as compared to a non-smoker.

- Drink a lot of water to flush nicotine from your system.

- Practise yoga and meditation for a healthy heart.

- Improve your diet. Eat a diet rich in fruits, vegetables and whole grains (breads, cereals and rice). Avoid fried food and meat (liver and kidney). Do not take egg yolk, butter and saturated fats.

- For cooking use sunflower or olive oil instead of butter and ghee.

- Use lemon or vinegar in salads for dressing.

- Reduce stress

- Stop worrying

- Control your blood pressure. Get your blood pressure checked once a week. In case of high blood pressure keep your weight normal, have low-fat calcium-rich diet, reduce the intake of salt, avoid alcoholic beverages and smoking.

- Switch to a low-fat diet to lower the cholesterol, build up in the body. Avoid foods high in sodium such as canned soups, canned vegetables, shellfish and pickled meals.

- Check diabetes if there are symptoms such as excessive thirst, excessive urination, constant weight loss, dehydration and weakness, leg cramps and blurred vision.

- Yogic postures such as *pranayama* and *shavasana* are beneficial exercises for a cardiovascular patient.

Insomnia

Insomnia is a sleep disorder in which the patient is unable to sleep. Sleeping pills, however, are effective for short-term treatment, but these become ineffective and can cause many side effects. There are several natural steps for inducing good sleep.

- Avoid stress. Choose a noiseless quiet place for sleep.

- Sleeping pills are a nightmare and interfere with the normal functioning of the brain causing poor sleep.

- For relaxation focus your mind on various organs of the body such as hands, feet, thighs, stomach, chest, shoulder, neck, face and forehead.

- Monitor your breathing. Place one hand on your stomach and the other on your chest. Deep breathing relaxes the muscles.

- High carbohydrate diet eaten before sleep increases serotonin (a brain chemical) that promotes sleep.

- Do not sleep more than required. A newborn baby requires sleep up to 18 hours a day. A 10-year-old child needs 9-10 hours sleep. An adult requires sleep between 7-8 hours. Sleep depends on an individual's requirement. Few people need 5-6 hours sleep whereas others of the same age group need up to 9-10 hours sleep. If you are unable to sleep, read a magazine or a book.

- Avoid stimulants such as coffee, colas and chocolates that contain caffeine.

- Take a warm bath before retiring to bed for good sleep.

- Try sex before sleep. Sexual activity help enhance sleep. Remember, if sex causes anxiety and problems, you will not enjoy good sleep.

- Acupressure treatment helps to induce a good sleep. Consult a naturopath to suggest a suitable treatment.

Menopause

Menopause is the time in a woman's life when her menstrual periods end. It is often called the 'change of life'. At menopause, the ovaries also stop producing egg. The completion of menopause marks the end of a woman's child bearing years.

Following are the symptoms of menopause:
- Hot flushes and sudden chills.
- Decrease in sexual desire.
- Vaginal dryness and loss of sex drive.
- Emotional distress.
- Insomnia (sleeping problems).
- Depression.
- Memory loss and sudden change of mood.

- Night sweating. Sometimes, the sweating is so high one may have to change the bed sheet.
- In case of vaginal bleeding consult a doctor immediately.

The following measures are beneficial during menopause:

- Regular exercise should be a part of daily life. Walking, jogging, bicycling, jumping rope, dancing, swimming or any other light exercise relieve menopausal disorders.
- More than 75% women usually have hot flushes due to body's response to lower estrogen levels, lasting between two to three minutes. During excretion of hot flushes, heat is produced in the body, the face reddens and there is excessive sweating.
- Nutrients can help control or completely eliminate hot flushes. Vitamin A is as effective as estrogen (recommended daily dose – 400 to 1200 international units). In case of night sweats, have two doses during the night after consulting the doctor.
- Learn meditation. Sit quietly, eyes closed to relax your mind.
- Alcohol triggers hot flushes. Similarly cut down caffeinated beverages that stimulate the production of the stress hormones and trigger hot flushes.
- Wear fibre clothes. Synthetic clothes trap heat and produce perspiration during hot flushes.
- Drink a lot of water or juice, especially after exercising.
- Eat small meals–minimum three meals a day. Even five to six small meals a day help the body to regulate the temperature easily.
- Vitamin B complex helps to reduce stress in menopausal women.
- The herb sage works very well if menopausal woman have hot flushes throughout the day and sweat during night. Drink sage tea.
- Hydrotherapy is very helpful for menopausal women. The body expels toxins during menstruation. When menstrual discharge decreases or stops, the body releases toxins through sweating or hot flushes. It is advised to have *sauna* (steam) bath to release toxins from the body. In case a sauna or steam bath is not possible, take a hot bath for 10-20 minutes a day.

- The herbs – valerian and lavender help in getting sound sleep. Take 300 to 500 milligrams valerian extract an hour before retiring to bed at night. Dab few drops of lavender essential oil on your pillow before sleep, which helps to get a sound sleep.

- Acupressure therapy relieves insomnia and anxiety in menopausal women. Stimulate pressure points on the feet for 1 to 3 minutes each with middle and index fingers.

- Women who have regular intercourse after menopause once a week or once a fortnight, have few or no hot flushes or night sweating as compared to those women who don't indulge in sexual intercourse at all. Having frequent sexual activity helps the drop in estrogen levels, which reduces hot flushes as the ovaries are stimulated.

- Vitamin E helps in case of vaginal dryness. It can also be used to massage the perineum. Various lubricants such as vaginal jelly, vegetable oil and unscented cream or oil can be used for vaginal dryness.

- Break open vitamin E capsules, mix with the lubricant and massage.

- Yoga aids relaxation and reduces stress. *Ekpada uttanasana* and *ek hasta bhujangasana* are recommended yoga exercises to be practised when a woman passes through the menopausal period.

Ek Hasta Bhujangasana

This is a posture of the leg supported by the arm. Sit on with palms resting on the floor. Keep the right leg straight on the floor and left leg resting on the left shoulder. Raise the hips upwards keeping the balance on both arms. Stay in this position for 5 to 6 minutes and lower the body on the floor.

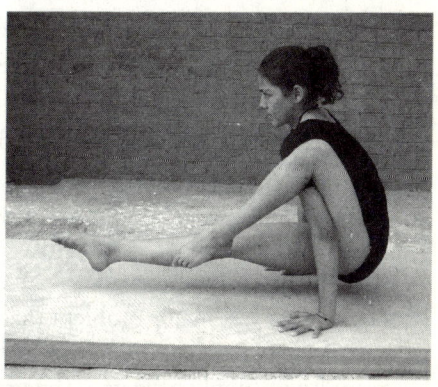

Ek Hasta Bhujangasana

Return to the initial sitting position. Rest for a while and repeat the posture 4 to 5 times.

Benefits

- Strengthens the abdominal muscles and fortifies the arms, wrists and hands.

Ek Pada Uttanasana

Lie down on your back with heels together. Let the body remain loose. Inhale slowly and raise the right leg upwards in a perpendicular position to the floor without straining, twisting or turning the hips and waist. Lower the leg on the floor exhaling. Rest for 6 to 8 seconds and repeat the exercise on the left leg.

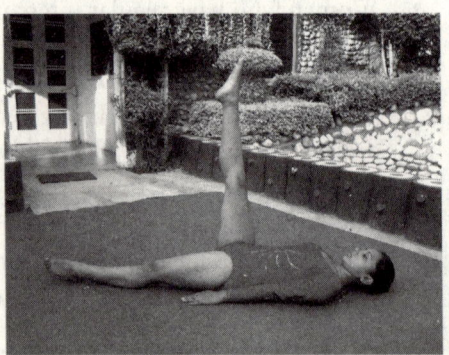

Ek Pada Uttanasana

Benefits

- Tones up the muscles of the sex glands and enhances the potentiality during menopausal period.
- Cures all menstrual disorders and white vaginal discharge.
- Tones up the muscles of the sex glands during menopause and enhances the potentiality in women, having lack of interest in sexual activity.
- Cures asthma and makes the hip joints flexible.
- Corrects the disorders of stomach and intestine, relieves wind troubles and gastric conditions of the digestive system.

Anaemia

Iron deficiency is a major problem that affects every one out of five women. Anaemia is a condition in which limited red blood cells have lesser ability to supply oxygen to the tissues resulting in weakness.

Symptoms of Anaemia

- Dizziness
- Loss of appetite
- Diarrhoea
- Abdominal pain
- Pale complexion
- Palpitation of the heart
- Shortness of breath
- Feeling of weakness
- Frequent headache

The blood needs iron to produce red cells. Women having insufficient iron in their diets or those who have heavy menstrual discharge may lack in desired levels of red blood cells or haemoglobin and the oxygen carrying protein in red blood cells. Women who feel tired and weak or have heavy or lengthy menstrual flow lasting for more than seven days or rectal bleeding should consult the doctor and improve their diet and lifestyle.

To examine if suffering from anaemia, press unpolished fingernail against the nail bed for few seconds, the area turns white and when stopped pressing the nail turns pink. However, a complete blood examination performed in a competent laboratory may confirm that a woman is anaemic. Remember, the loss of blood during periods must be replaced by fresh blood produced in the bone marrow, which requires enough iron in the diet of a woman.

Blood is the fluid circulating through blood vessels containing red blood cells, platelets and a pale yellowish liquid known as plasma, which acts as a fluid medium for the suspension of blood cells, transports dissolved nutrients to the tissues, carries waste products from tissues to the organs. The red blood cells contain haemoglobin, a red pigment of the blood. They also produce proteins called antibodies, which fight infection.

Types of Anaemia

Type	Effects
Sickle-cell Anaemia	A chemical abnormality of haemoglobin in the blood cells. More common in children causing jaundice, thin arms and a protruding abdomen as a result of lack of blood circulation in the body. To treat sickle-cell anaemia, blood transfusions are given to restore red cells. Good nutrition, plenty of fluids and vitamins help to improve the condition. A female suffering from sickle-cell anaemia needs a genetic counselling before conceiving.
Deficient anaemia	Caused due to lack of a substance necessary for the formation of blood.
Pernicious anaemia	Results from vitamin B12 deficiency. Women suffering from pernicious anaemia should take vitamin B12 throughout their life.
Iron-deficiency anaemia	Caused due to the loss of blood. It can be treated by blood transfusion or giving iron pills to produce red blood cells.
Congenital anaemia	Occurs in women born with defective blood. The blood cells are destroyed in the body.
Hemolytic anaemia	It is caused by diseased cells in the body, which run in families due to inherited defects in the blood.

Some home remedies to cure anaemia are given below:

• Have iron-rich food including whole grains such as barley, oats, beans, peas, seeds and nuts, soyabeans, sesame seeds, soups, fruits and green vegetables.

- Calcium rich foods supply iron to the body. Remember, dairy products decrease iron absorption in anaemic women.

- Vitamin C is acidic and helps the body to absorb iron contents. Squeeze the juice of a lemon into a glass of water and drink before meals or take vitamin C in consultation with the doctor (required daily dose – 1,000 to 2,000 milligrams with each meal).

- Alcoholic beverages (wine and beer) deplete the body of vitamin B complex and minerals that worsen anaemia.

- Reduce the intake of sugar, which depletes the body of vitamin B complex.

- Avoid having caffeinated products such as coffee, black tea, soda and chocolate in your daily diet, as it depletes the body of vitamin B complex.

- If anaemia results from iron deficiency, iron pills are suggested. In case anaemia is associated with vitamin B12, deficiency vitamins are administered through injections.

- Recommended yogic postures for anaemia patients are *sarvangasana* and *paschimottanasana*.

Constipation and Indigestion

Constipation is a condition in which the bowel does not rid itself of the waste as readily as usual. Constipated people do not have regular bowel movements, may have pain over the colon and also rectal bleeding. The following solutions relieve constipation:

- Take fibre in the diet. A daily consumption of 20 to 35 gm of dietary fibre is required for adults. Green peas, apple, bran, cereal, oatmeal, dried beans and nuts are rich source of fibre.

- Exercise is good for the bowels to combat constipation.

- 8 to 10 glasses of water should be taken daily.

- Improve your bowel habits. The most natural time to go to the toilet is early morning hours. Sit on the toilet for ten minutes even if you don't feel the urge to relieve yourself.

- Beware of certain foods including milk to relieve constipation. Sometimes milk may cause diarrhoea. Avoid foods such as beans, cauliflower and cabbage – all these tend to produce gas.
- Avoid large meals that distend the digestive tract and worsen constipation.
- Aloevera juice, dandelion root and plantain seeds are very useful to treat constipation.
- Have a glass of lukewarm water with lemon juice with ½ teaspoon of honey added in the morning.
- Olive, canola and other monounsaturated and polyunsaturated oils act as digestive lubricant helping out in relieving constipation.
- Massage your colon, the final section of the digestive tract, where constipation takes place, using the fingertips. Massage the right side of the abdominal area moving in a circular motion till the hands reach above the belly button. Continue to massage down to your hips in the same way.
- '*Triphala*' is a laxative which helps in relieving constipation. Take one tablespoon thrice a day.
- Yogic postures recommended to relieve constipation are – *mayurasana, supta vajrasana, padmasana, shallabhasana, bakasana, halasana, ek pada uttanasana, ourdhva paschim-uttanasana* and *matsyendrasana*

Mayurasana (the peacock posture)

Kneel on the ground, knees apart, palms flat on the floor, fingers pointing towards the feet and place the elbows under the abdomen.

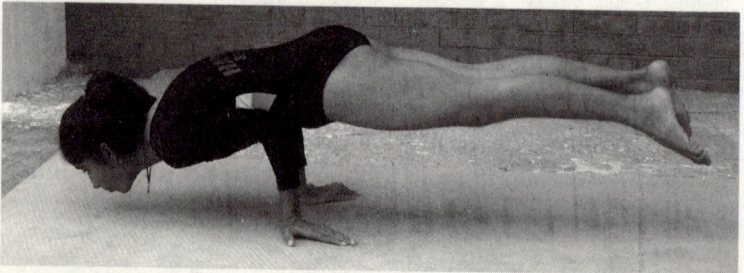

Mayurasana

Lean forward to touch the floor with your forehead and stretch out the legs behind. Raise the head and body parallel to the ground staying balanced on the arms. Stay in this position as long as possible comfortably. Return to the initial position and lie down on the stomach. Relax for sometime and repeat the posture for 2-3 times.

Benefits

- Relieves chronic constipation and increases the supply of blood to the digestive organs.
- Tones up the abdominal and forearm muscles.
- Regenerates energy in the body. Brings the body into equilibrium.

Bakasana (the crow posture)

Put the right feet on the thigh of the left leg and left feet on the thigh of the right leg. Place the palms on the floor near the feet. Raise hips and head, resting knees on the upper arms. Sway the body forward and raise the body off the floor balancing on the hands.

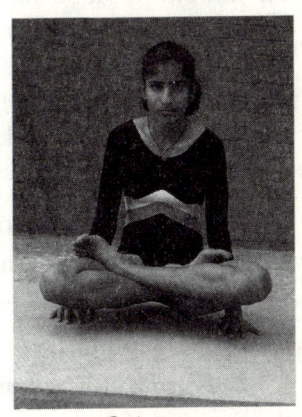

Bakasana

Benefits

- Strengthens the muscles of the arms, wrists and shoulders.
- Provides strength, confidence and improves concentration.

Diabetes

Diabetes is a serious disease having the following symptoms:

- Increased thirst and dry mouth
- Frequent urination
- Increased appetite
- Vomiting and diarrhoea
- Blurred vision
- Rapid or irregular heart beat

- Dizziness and fatigue
- Weight loss
- Urinary tract infections
- Decreased consciousness leading to coma

If the disease exceeds for more than a week, consult a physician for diagnosis. Excess sugar in the blood damages the arteries and veins and can lead to fatal heart disease. Diabetes can also cause kidney disease, eye problems and can damage the nerves of the lower limbs and other parts of the body.

Nearly 10% of the diabetics suffer from the disease because of the attack on the immune system. The pancreas stops producing insulin, a hormone which regulates glucose in the body. As a result the amount of blood sugar or glucose rises in the blood stream leading to diabetes which ushers blood sugar (glucose) out of the blood stream and into the cells of the body. Insulin injections are administered to cure diabetes, which sometimes begins in childhood causing a lifetime insulin dependency. Such type of diabetes is called 'Juvenile diabetes' which is usually diagnosed before the age of 20.

The following home remedies are advised to treat diabetes:

- Avoid cow's milk. It may cause an intense allergic reaction.
- Avoid all foods containing grains.
- Reduce sugar intake.
- Fatty acids such as flaxseed oil help repair the cellular damage.
- Exercising for 15 minutes in the morning and evening eliminates the risk of developing diabetes by 25% and normalises blood sugar.
- Acupressure therapy heals diabetes. Press the following pressure points on the body for two to three seconds each:
  1. Above the bulge of the ankle bone.
  2. The hollow area midway between the ankle bone and the back of the ankle.
  3. One centimetre below the inside of the ankle bone.
  4. Four inches below the navel in a vertical line running down in the middle of the body.

5.   Above the navel, between the navel and the lower edge of sternum, outside the elbow at the end of the skin's crease.

6.   Inside of the elbow on the outer edge of the ridge of tendons.

7.   In the web between thumb and index fingers.

8.   On the crease of the wrist closest to the palms on the inside of the radial artery.

• Yogic postures such as *ourdhva paschimottanasana* and *ardha matsyendrasana* help cure diabetes.

Ardha Matsyendrasana

Sit on the floor. Straighten the body stretching both the legs in front in a parallel position. Breath normally. Fold the left leg. Take right leg on the other side of the left leg and with the left hand hold the right foot or ankle. The right knee should be as near as possible to the left armpit. Turn the body to the right. Twist the back and then the neck as far as possible. Stay in this position for 6-8 seconds and return to the initial position. Repeat this on the other side also.

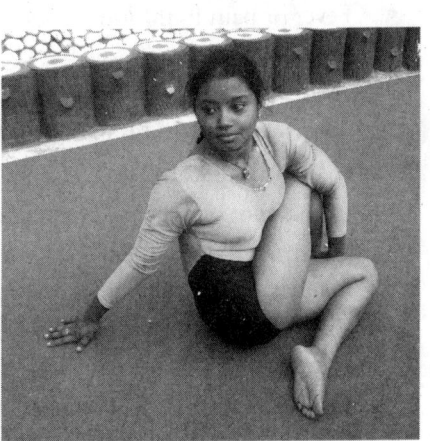

Ardha Matsyendrasana

Benefits

• Leaves a beneficial effect on the pancreas, adrenal, thyroid and sex glands.

• Activates the muscles of the stomach, abdomen, intestine, kidneys, spleen, liver and spinal cord.

• Energises and strengthens the body.

• Good for diabetics.

Kidney Disorders

Kidney disorders, mostly stone in kidneys are common among women. In 70 to 75% of cases kidney stones are composed of calcium oxalate crystals, whereas in approximately 10% cases, they are made of uric acid crystals. Following symptoms are seen in case of kidney stones:

- Severe pain which is not relieved by drinking large amount of fluids.
- Pain doesn't disappear in spite of taking pain killers.
- Blood in the urine
- Inability to pass urine
- Fever or pain in the kidneys or in the lower back near the end of the rib cage.

Following are the natural ways to treat kidney stones:

- id fatty foods, fibre foods, white sugar and white flour.
- ..... eating leafy green vegetables that can cause kidney stones.
- Drink a lot of water approximately 6-8 glasses a day.
- Vitamins D and B6 and minerals such as calcium and magnesium prevent the formation of stones.
- Exercise helps keep calcium from draining out of the bones with urine.
- Drink 2 to 3 glasses of orange, grapefruit and tomato juice every day to keep the right pH balance.
- Have at least 8 glasses of water a day to prevent the formation of uric acid stones.
- Yoga helps in treating kidney disorders. Recommended yogic postures are *dhanurasana, ushtrasana, chakrasana, karnapidasana, bhujangasana, paschimottanasana, shalabhasana* and *ardha matsyendrasana.*